Praise for HUNDRED PERCENT CHANCE

"Brown examines the rigors of cancer treatment in his candid debut memoir. . . This intimate, passionate chronicle of recovery will appeal to those who've battled cancer."

– Publishers Weekly

"While memoirs of surviving disease are plenty, *Hundred Percent Chance* stands apart through its genuine humor and unflinching portrayal of both the physical and psychological struggles that accompany a diagnosis of disease. . . . This memoir's focus on the tiny moments that ultimately shape and define a life, are particularly poignant and engrossing."

– The BookLife Prize 2019

"Brown's writing is lively and lyrical, with moments of intense description offset by humorous ones. . . . For those interested in seeing the toll leukemia can take on a young, healthy person, Brown's account offers the details in searing prose. An intense, deftly composed cancer narrative."

– Kirkus Reviews

"Robert K. Brown's medical memoir *Hundred Percent Chance* is larger than life without trying to be. . . . While the content of the book is raw, brutal, and honest, it is Brown's lively, rebellious attitude — and understanding that he was lucky to go into remission so quickly and to receive such excellent care — that makes this book a triumph. . . . *Hundred Percent Chance* is an inspiring, provocative memoir about dealing with cancer that maintains its sense of humor when the going gets rough."

– Foreword Clarion Reviews

"Brown's straightforward, unpretentious writing style is compelling and brutally honest. The use of present tense, first person, amplifies the effect. His wry sense of humor is both endearing and heartbreaking. . . . Regardless of one's personal experience with cancer or critical illness, these pages relate an essential human experience: the struggle to survive against the odds. This universal theme will resonate with almost any reader."

– BlueInk Review

"A realistic, in-your-face honest and down-to-earth memoir about the rigors of treating and surviving cancer, handled with both intimacy and concern."

– IndieReader

"Robert takes the reader inside the world of AML – an unexpected journey of diagnosis, treatment, and survival of a subset of AML that he was not supposed to survive. But, he did. . . . Within these pages you'll discover and come to understand Robert's mindset. Simply, but painfully it was: I will survive. No questioning, no heroics – just, I'm going to live. *Hundred Percent Chance: A Memoir* is an opportunity to live and feel the fear, the discouragement, the pain, the exhaustion, the struggle, the determination, the elation of surviving a monster."

**– Michael Copley, National Chairman, Beat AML,
The Leukemia & Lymphoma Society**

"The writing is gorgeous, almost lyrical, and it captures the voice of a young man in the '90s, one filled with strength and eloquence. *Hundred Percent Chance: A Memoir* evokes powerful emotions in readers – hope and despair, joy and frustration, love and pain – but the throbbing life within the protagonist, a life that permeates the narrative, will keep readers turning the pages."

– Readers' Favorite

"Brown has a gift for weaving life arcs in and out of his writing. He captures the urgency of an unforeseen emergency as nimbly as the grinding march of a long, degrading chemo run. Important characters in his battle are allowed to shine and then recede as people often do in our lives. His story is presented in a dynamic flow of scene and feeling rather than an abrupt hopscotch from one square to the next. *Hundred Percent Chance* is both honest and present in its struggle, its naiveté and its determination."

– Paul Miller, author of *Vantage Point*

"Stories like these are invaluable to patients, their families, and medical care professionals because they flesh out the realities of all aspects of cancer treatment... Author Robert Brown has given the world a gift by sharing his words."

– Judge, 27th Annual Writer's Digest Self-Published Book Awards

HUNDRED PERCENT CHANCE

A Memoir

Robert K. Brown

Published by 3/3 Press
8725 Columbine Rd – Unit 46362
Eden Prairie, MN 55344

ISBN 978-1-7331590-0-5

www.hundredpercentchance.com

Cover Design by Melissa Williams Design

For Cindy and Anne

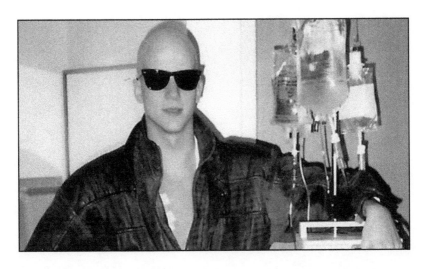

Trying to look cool in the midst of chemotherapy, summer 1990.

PROLOGUE

I had leukemia. I had it and now I don't and that should be that. Only it's not. It's a memory that won't go away. Not a haunting memory, not a slow-motion replay of a rear-end collision where you find yourself clenching your arms against the seat, looking back over your shoulder for the too-fast car that isn't there. No. Leukemia is vague with occasional flashes of coherence. It is a constant hum.

During the summer of 1992, not even two full years after my last stay in the hospital, I would be sitting on the back porch with Dad and Jane – all of us sharing sections from the thick Sunday paper, arguing over who would get the comics first – when a palpable memory would surprise me. I would not be expecting it, and the memories were still so fresh.

Perhaps one of my legs had fallen asleep, or the coffee had cooled slightly, a tight bitter taste. Something: a glint of sunlight reflecting off Green Lake down the hill. *Anything.* There would be a sudden flash in my brain, telling me that the tingling sensation was *exactly* the way my legs felt after those first seven weeks at the University of Washington Medical Center: emaciated, weak, thin, practically useless. They wobbled when I tried walking up the stairs after I'd finally made it back home. That feeling would come crashing down around me. I would be sitting in a comfortable chair on the back porch with my parents, warm morning sun pouring through the windows, good coffee, all of that, but suddenly my legs are once again beyond weak and tired, a memory of such aching, exhausted pain.

I'd stare through the newspaper. And then I'd be tasting the chemo again, tasting it bad like it was during those earliest weeks. Maybe I'd feel a quick rush, a hot spurt in my veins of something, I don't know what or why, and I'm flat on my back again, in this claustrophobic subterranean hospital room, one of many faceless nurses standing at my side. She is pushing iodine into my bloodstream so the CAT scan images will be clearer, all because of mystery fevers out of nowhere, again and again, this time well into my final round of chemotherapy. Only now my doctors and nurses and family and everyone else are all but certain — *shh, don't tell anyone* — that the solution to the mystery is that my fevers are starting from somewhere inside my skull.

These were real. Tangible. It doesn't do them justice to simply call them "memories." The colors would be so clear, the smells, the sounds, the heat in my veins, that nasty metallic taste, and then quiet fucking tears that would need to be blinked away before Dad or Jane might notice.

The constant hum of leukemia would transform into a brief shout.

Pay attention, it says. *Do not forget me. I can make your body remember, even if your mind wants to forget.*

As if I could.

I'm talking with Mom, in that same hazy summer after graduating from Carleton, a couple of years after everything. We'd be talking in the kitchen at the new house her and Paul had recently moved into up the hill near Fairwood. She's working on a grocery list, standing in front of the refrigerator with a small note pad, opening and closing cupboards almost at random, adding more items to her list. I'm leaning up against the corner by the double sinks, swishing a glass of water around, listening to the ice clank against the sides, asking her what she thinks about insurance. We would talk about this fairly often after graduation. It concerns me, my inability to find medical insurance with such an ominous pre-existing condition. COBRA won't last forever. I'm an adult, now. Didn't get into grad school. Don't have a full-time job. What am I supposed to do if I can't find a "real" job? I sure as hell can't afford insurance premiums if I keep waiting tables or working shitty office temp jobs in downtown Seattle. The clock is ticking.

I'm not even paying much attention to what I'm saying, just random questions for her to field. She's *The Mom*, the solid, strong businesswoman. She knows about these things. But suddenly she's crying. Real tears, running fast, and they make me uncomfortable. "I'm sorry," she says. "It still surprises me how quickly they come. Just when I think I have it under control..."

"I'm sorry..."

"Don't be sorry, Robert. It's me."

Her memories, I think, are sometimes even stronger than mine. Or perhaps they are simply that much more painful. More painful to be on the outside looking in, unable to do anything but worry, unable to dab peroxide on a skinned knee. Leukemia is one thing that a mother cannot kiss and make better.

When I was in the hospital, both sets of parents encouraged me to take notes, keep a journal, anything to help me to remember what we were going through. There were so many free hours, so many days where I couldn't do anything but move from my bed to my bathroom and back again.

Just jot down some details, they'd suggested. *Take your time. Write things down.*

My sister's best friend had given me a new Sony Walkman during my first month in the hospital, one of many thoughtful gifts from many early visitors. It was an upgraded model, with an additional button to press that would allow me to speak into a small microphone at the bottom and record anything onto a blank cassette tape.

"I know you've been tired," Sharon had said. "But you can still speak into this if you want, you know. You don't even have to write. Just preserve the memories."

Another acquaintance — a long-time friend and former secretary of my mother's — had also been shopping. Everybody, it seemed, was on the same page. Working together to get me thinking about the words I should be putting to paper. She'd picked out a hard cover notebook with a marbled blue cover and clean blank pages to go along with a gorgeous Waterman pen, blue, medium point.

I appreciated all of it. *Really.* But I was always so fucking tired.

"Besides," I'd told them, individually, collectively, "How could I possibly forget? This isn't the sort of experience that's likely to fade from memory anytime soon."

"No, no," they would respond. "That's not what we meant. *Of course* you'll never forget that you had leukemia. But you might forget the name of one particular doctor. Not all of them, but maybe one or two. Or the man who worked in Food Services, the one with the vast personal library of movies on VHS tape, black-and-white classics, mostly, bringing a new one for you to enjoy every day with your lunch. You might forget what he looks like, his name, the different movies he'd brought. Even the way your chest felt, remember, when it was swollen with blood? When you couldn't stop bleeding after your Hickman catheter was put in? These things. These specific moments are the kinds of details that might vanish forever."

"Oh. That's it? Nothing to worry about," I'd told them

I was twenty, twenty-one years old, as confident as one can be after enduring weeks of chemotherapy and complications.

"Don't worry," I'd said. "I'll remember everything."

Wrong.

I remember that I survived. I remember only a few of the most lucid dreams. Names have slowly disappeared behind a dark wall of fog. Specifics, for the most part, elude me. Or maybe it's just that I haven't made sufficient attempts to dredge my memory yet.

One of my first doctors at the University of Washington Medical Center — young, tall, square-jawed and ruggedly handsome, like he'd stepped straight out of central casting for some popular weeknight drama — had told my parents that one of the likely side-effects of my steady diet of drugs could very well be memory loss.

"We'll be prescribing them primarily to fight infection," he'd said. "That's our immediate, short term goal. In addition to providing his body with some much-needed protection against infection, they might well do a number on his memory. He may forget. Might not be such a bad trade-off, no? Some things are better left unremembered."

This, then, will be my belated attempt to remember, so many years later. *I will write.* I will chase my memories, tackling them from behind if necessary, capturing them on paper. Hopefully they'll progress in a linear, chronological fashion, but no guarantees. Memories like Jackson Pollack. A burst of color there, a dribble of paint, more splashes in the corner because that red reminds me of this shade of crimson, and before long there's a complete picture: the story of my leukemia.

CHAPTER 1

Here is how it all begins: in darkness. In silence. Colors slowly bleed in from the sides, an out-of-focus jumble of greens and blues and whites. The camera sharpens. It's a panoramic view, a wide countryside. The hills are damp with recent rain. Imagine a camera slowly panning across miles of vibrant green farmland. Roll soundtrack: low horns and a rippling piano. Or, better, an instrumental from the eighties, something like New Order's *Elegia*. Something preposterously British.

An old farmhouse passes by the corner of your eye. A broken stone wall. A light mist hangs in the air, as if the evening is unable to decide whether to return to the rain from earlier in the day or to just let the clouds disappear into the night. There's still some light left, but it's fading fast. The camera stops to focus on a group of white buildings. They're planted along the crest of a gentle green hill. The buildings look a little out of place: very modern and angular, surrounded by the rustic countryside, acres of multi-colored farmland and hundred-year-old thatched roofs.

It is a university campus, this collection of buildings, with a visible central path running from north to south, like a spinal cord. The students will call it exactly this, *the Spine*, as they walk from one end of the university to another. The buildings are close together, a compact design. The setting sun breaks through a gap in the clouds, reflecting off a long row of dormitory windows on the south end of the campus. The camera continues to zoom in, closer, slowly, closer, until the upper two-thirds of the screen are filled by an open ground-floor window.

The imaginary camera pushes through the curtains. The room is small. There is a narrow bed against the near wall to the right, and a kind of combination desk/bookshelf/wardrobe on the other. The room is no more than six feet or eight feet wide. A door is centered in the wall immediately opposite the window. There is a small sink and mirror next to the door, sandwiched in the tiny space between the end of the wardrobe and the interior wall.

It's not a sink you use for cooking. It's much too small for that. Some nights you come home late after drinking with your mates, and you've flopped down onto your bed, staring at the spinning spinning spinning white ceiling, wishing it would stop moving. You know you're not going to be able to stumble all the way down the hall to the common bathroom. The walls would probably be lurching from side-to-side anyway, taunting you. It's understood, right, that you maybe shouldn't have had those last two or three pints. But the boys were buying, and you were drinking, and now it's a little late to regret the fun you'd had.

The small sink in the corner is useful for brushing your teeth twice a day — for checking your hair before you go out at night, and for quick standing "showers" when you've overslept before class — but it's *especially* useful for emergency late-night vomiting.

There is a young man sitting at the desk in this narrow, nondescript dorm room. He's pushed the chair back onto two legs, so that it rests up against the bed immediately behind him. His eyes are closed, but the leg he's used to push off from the desk vibrates with nervous energy. Headphones are tucked into his ears, snaking down to a bright yellow Walkman in his lap. His head moves in time, almost imperceptibly, with the fading soundtrack.

This is his room. His story.

No. That's not right. This is *my* room. *This is my story.*

I am wearing shorts and a sweaty tee-shirt underneath an oversized (and well-soaked) Pendle College sweatshirt. My shoes are kicked into some corner or another. I don't really care. I've just returned from a short run. There is a winding two lane road that circles around the entire campus, just about a mile, a perfect loop for running. It's been an incredibly convenient route this past handful of months. I'm able to squeeze in a quick run any time of the day. I'll just lift up my window, crawl outside, and start running. Most days I'll double or even triple the loop. Headphones securely fastened, rain seeping into my arms and shoulders, sharp breaths cutting through the mist.

I'm in decent shape. Better than average. I've been working at it since I'd first come to Lancaster last October, the almost compulsory "junior year abroad" from my idyllic Midwest liberal arts college. I'm probably as fit as I've ever been, between regularly hitting the weights at the gym, practice and games with the volleyball club, early morning or late afternoon runs, not to mention a short-lived attempt to join the crew team (because what could be a more stereotypically British experience, I'd thought, than rowing along glassy rivers in and around Lancaster).

So I'm in pretty reasonably great shape, right, but I am absolutely *exhausted* after only a single lap outside my window. After only one stupid fucking mile.

I'm not sucking wind, not out of breath, but I'm still categorically wiped out. Beyond lethargic: I'm dead on my feet. It doesn't make any sense. That's why I'm sitting at my desk, leaning back onto two chair legs, trying to figure out what's wrong.

It's been at least the past few days — or maybe closer to a week, I don't know — that I've been feeling more beaten down than normal. Nothing obvious, nothing specific, just steadily higher levels of crushing fatigue. I figure it's just how it gets sometimes, late winter, when you can feel a cold approaching, all scratchy throat and tired eyes and limbs. That's not to say that it is a cold, or the flu, or anything. It's probably just my body getting so sick and tired of the non-stop rain and fog and darkness, of a sun that sets so early in the day — especially this far north — that it's felt like weeks since I've last had so much as a glimpse of the sun.

And it *is* late February, too. I get that.

Plus, I haven't had the best sleeping habits, either, since I've been here. Lots of late nights out drinking and carousing with the boys.

This shitty feeling could be anything. A warning shot, I suppose, telling me to get some real rest, to give my body some time to recover or else I'll end up sniffling and coughing until things finally start to warm up a bit in March.

I know it could be any number of perfectly reasonable, perfectly rational things. My quick evening run was an attempt to push back. My show of strength.

Look, body, I'm in charge here. Understand? We're going to get outside, even if it's cold and wet, and we're going to run. And we are absolutely not going to whine or complain or get sick. You got that?

It was supposed to be three laps, three miles, but I'm back here at my desk after only one. I'm still tired, dragging, and feeling even worse than before I'd gone out. Some show of strength. My body has called my bluff.

I look down at my legs, twisting them around so I can see the backs of my calves and thighs. Then I look a little more closely at my arms and hands. It's not good. The front of the chair falls to the ground. Momentum carries my arms over to my desk. I reach out for my journal, flipping through pages of notes and sketches and unfinished poems until I find a blank page near the end. I uncap my pen, then take a deep breath. Several deep breaths. My eyes are closed. I'm deliberating. Delaying. Do I really want to write this down? I'm afraid, I think, that putting these thoughts to paper will somehow give them substance. It will lend them a permanence that I'm not sure I'm ready to face.

I guess it doesn't really matter. I'm feeling what I'm feeling, whether it's written in my journal or not. Simply writing something down doesn't make it any more or less true.

19 Feb 1990

A bruise on the outside of my right calf; a bruise that swells up around the ring finger knuckle on my right hand; a couple of bruises on the upper back part of both legs; a healthy bruise on my waist where Si Shaw pinched me (at least that one is explainable). A new bruise, strong, on my left foot. Small red spots on both feet that crawl a little ways up my shins. A sore on the inside of my mouth.

I don't know what is going on here, and I'm scared. Not scared enough to go to the doctor and say "oh, look, I've got a bunch of Mystery Bruises," but scared enough to write this down. I don't know. Maybe it's nothing. But my body is falling apart on me and I don't like it. Shit. This is just for the record: as of 19 Feb 1990 I am frightened because things are happening to me that I can't explain away.

My mind is racing. My heart.

I try thinking of diseases that make people bruise easily. The only word that comes to mind is hemophilia. Weak blood or something? That's hemophilia, right? Or is it anemia?

Fuck.

I don't know. I don't what it is, don't know what it might be other than something bad. My legs are still warm from my run. I rub my hands across the unblemished tops of my thighs. Inspiration comes quickly. I know, now, what to do about the uncertainty and doubt: a test.

I could test myself, test whether these bruises really have been happening so easily. Simple enough. I push back from my desk, stretching out my right leg, making sure to flex. I tense up, toe pointed. Calf and quad both tighten. I make a fist. A good one. I focus on a spot on the middle of my thigh, a couple of inches below my shorts. I pound it. Twice. Three times. I use all sides of my fist, pounding with the bottom, then with my knuckles. I crook my pointer finger out to make a tiny knob. Again and again and again. One last time for good measure.

See, now, see? It makes absolute sense to punch my thigh multiple times — good, hard hits — and if it doesn't bruise tomorrow then I'm clearly okay. Clearly. This journal entry will become something to laugh about with the boys next weekend. A joke for the ages. My leg throbs red. It hurts, but I'm smiling as I stand up, thinking how clever I've been. This will be a good test. One day is the deadline. Twenty-four hours. I will give it one day to turn into a bruise.

This time tomorrow I'll know for sure.

CHAPTER 2

I wake up, groggy, around noon. Twelve or thirteen hours of sleep and I'm still tired. I've already missed both of my classes for the day. And I don't really care. I know I should have at least been able to get up in time for my Jane Austen class, which started maybe five minutes ago, but my bed is supremely comfortable. So warm and cozy. I could maybe lounge around under the covers for another several hours, plenty of time before I meet up with Simon to head over to volleyball practice later.

It is too tempting. Instead, I force myself to kick my legs out from underneath my comforter, wipe the sleep from the corners of my eyes, and shuffle over to the small sink in the corner of my room.

Cold water, cold washcloth, toothbrush and toothpaste. Swish. Spit. Blood.

Blood?

Another spit and this time it is all blood, no toothpaste. I tuck my thumbs underneath my top lip and lift up while squinting into the mirror. Blood pours out of my gums, running over my teeth. Shit. I've been brushing my teeth too hard, it seems. I guess this is what happens after spending so much time in England. All my mates have crappy teeth, you know? This must be what happens here.

I do not put two and two together. No light bulb moments for me here. There is no immediate association between what I'm seeing in the mirror and what I wrote about last night. It does not occur to me that there might be a relationship between them — or that perhaps this would have been a far better test.

My gums bleed throughout the day. They bleed while I devour a late lunch of a ham and cheese toasty with crisps (*not chips*) at the Junior Common Room. I can't really taste the blood in my food. I wash everything down with a tall glass of water. Volleyball practice is a sluggish, stupid waste of time, with frequent breaks to jog over to the water fountain to stay hydrated. And to discreetly spit out more blood, of course.

We're at the JCR at some point later in the evening, my regular after-dinner entertainment with the boys, enjoying multiple pints of beer between multiple rounds of pool. I remember that it was about this time yesterday that I'd come back from my run. I'm supposed to check my leg for bruising. I'm skeptical, because nothing has shown up throughout the day. This needs to be official, though, so I beg off from my next game of pool with Wayne.

The bathroom is empty, thankfully. I lock myself into the nearest stall and nervously pull down my jeans. I don't know why I'm worried. It should be fine. The light kind of sucks here, all flickering fluorescents, but it's the best I've got. I'm focused, careful, deliberate. I need to do this right. I need to be very thorough.

There's nothing.

The other bruises I'd written about in my journal — the myriad mystery bruises — can still be found pretty much everywhere I look. There's even some slight swelling around the pinky knuckle of my right hand after a stinger of a spike during practice earlier. The important one, though, the one I'd tried to create for myself isn't there.

Good. This is very good news.

* * *

There is a certain sameness to my time at Lancaster, a familiar and welcome repetition. Another night follows, another night spent at the JCR playing pool with Simon and Wayne and maybe a handful of other friends. It's early enough to still have a few other people hanging out reading or talking, playing pinball, sitting at the bar with a pint of ale. Faces I recognize if I don't know their names. There's a girl on the couch near the jukebox reading a thick textbook while sipping what looks to be a cider. Her name is Kristi, I think, or maybe Kirsten. Krista? I don't remember.

It's important to me, even feeling low, to be out with the boys. It's always a great time. Wayne has this cassette tape we've listened to countless times since I've been here. It's hilarious, this raunchy bit of comedy from Dudley Moore and Peter Cook, an improv radio show performed as these absolutely drunk-off-their-rockers characters they'd created, Derek and Clive. I'm sure they were legitimately drunk when they did these bits. They had to be. It's radio, though, so it's hard to tell.

The boys and I would come stumbling home from a night at the JCR, or from trying pints at some of the other colleges further up the Spine — the long central path that runs from Pendle College at very nearly the south end of campus up through various academic buildings and open courtyards to the north — and we'd all pile into Wayne's room well after closing time. He'd pop the tape into his cassette player and we'd play some of our favorite parts, mostly these ridiculously over-the-top conversations they had, simultaneously serious and ludicrous. Our laughter was contagious.

One of the funniest bits, the one that would have us doubled over, started with a riff about a non-stop disco dancer, and then somehow pivoted to this sing-songy improvisation about how one of their fathers has cancer. It's obviously ludicrous from the beginning. It picks up steam, heading downhill as they try to outdo one another as small children might. It's hilariously inappropriate, making light of such a serious subject.

And so we somehow find ourselves several pints into the night, the quality of our pool games getting progressively worse, finding more and more humor in the moment. It's mostly just us in the JCR anyway. Why not recreate our own little Derek and Clive scenes?

"I've got cancer of that shot," Wayne says to me, after I pocket a tough shot down the length of the table. When I miss the much easier follow-up, I complain about having cancer of my pool cue.

"I've got cancer of both of your ugly mugs," Simon says from the other table.

I'm fading fast. When it's Wayne's turn to shoot I rest against the now-unused pinball machine. I'm utterly exhausted. At the same time, it's so much fun here with my mates, and the laughter is such a tonic for how lousy I've been feeling this week, that I don't want to call it an early night. I'll stay out as late as I can tonight, periodically wiping my teeth with my tongue so the blood doesn't show.

Kristi/Kirsten/Krista has set her book down on the couch next to her. She's glaring across the room at us. "That's not funny, you know," she says, as we laugh at Jim's cancerously bad break. "That's not funny at all. There are people with cancer. You shouldn't make jokes."

"Bollocks," Wayne says. "I've got cancer of their cancer!"

"Really hilarious. Really mature. I hope nobody you know ever has cancer. It's not funny." She stuffs her book violently into her backpack, then gives all of us a measured glance before stomping off.

CHAPTER 3

I wake up twice during the night. The first time I'm shivering. Frozen. My comforter is tucked underneath my neck. My knees are balled up around my chest. Goosebumps raise the hair on my arms and legs.

Why is it so cold?

The second time is the opposite. I'm sweltering. Boiling. The comforter has been thrown to the floor. My tee-shirt is damp, as are my sheets, both drenched in sweat. It is a restless night. My mouth is dry when morning finally comes.

The kitchen on our floor is down the hall a few doors from mine, just past the common bathroom. It is early Saturday morning, and none of my floor mates are up yet. I pad down the hall, barefoot, in my underwear and a sort of fresh tee-shirt that's at least dry, if not particularly clean.

I'm hoping to find some leftover orange juice from the other day. I can't remember if I'd finished it or not. There it is, though, tucked into the crowded refrigerator door: a small, half-empty bottle of OJ. I finish it in a few gulps. After rinsing out the empty glass bottle, I set it upside down next to the sink to dry.

Outside, the morning drips wet and gray. The skies are heavy with charcoal clouds. Winds blow down from the north. I'm smiling, now, as I look out across the hills.

Today, I tell myself, *is the day I will get better.* There's nothing like a rainy Saturday for staying indoors all day, slurping up chicken noodle soup, drinking orange juice, and reading and resting. *Today is a perfect day to mend this battered body.*

The morning air is crisp and clean. I'm content.

I stop to use the bathroom on the way back to my room. I am still exhausted and feverish, I know, maybe a little wobbly standing above the toilet, but even still — it's impossible to deny what I see. My urine is bloody. No, that's not accurate. It's not so much that my urine is bloody as it is that I'm just straight up peeing blood.

What the …?

As far as I can tell there's no urine at all, just a steady stream of blood coming out of my body. The toilet water swirls red.

I shuffle back to my room. My left hand drags against the wall. I lock my door behind me. Not that anyone will be up for hours anyway, nor can I imagine Simon or Wayne knocking down my door, but I'm in need of some of that vaunted British privacy.

I glance at the clock on my desk: 7:52 AM. I'm trying to remember what I could have possibly done the day before that would have left me so utterly exhausted. There's nothing. There's no reason for this fatigue. There are no bruises on the top of my right thigh, either. Almost like a reflex, now, I run my tongue over my teeth and taste blood.

I will absolutely do something about this, I tell myself, crawling back into bed, eyes too heavy to keep open any longer, too tired to even finish my train of thought.

It's another couple of hours before I wake with a start. My window is fogged up. I open it about halfway and smell the cool air, thick and wet. On my desk, next to the window, is a crowded jumble of papers and books, pens, empty coffee cups, loose change. My journal is slim and black. It sits on a mostly empty corner of my desk. I lean up against the windowsill and thumb through the pages. I'm looking for that last entry, about three quarters of the way through the book. I'd written a note to myself, not even a week ago, a list of symptoms that I was ready to ignore. Should I add one more?

This is all wrong, I tell myself. *You know this is so very wrong.* With that, I am out the door, rushing back to the bathroom. I am still not convinced. I am still looking for more evidence. There is one simple way to prove that what happened earlier this morning was a delusion, nothing more than a bad, bloody dream.

Another test: my bladder burns from the half-bottle of orange juice from earlier. *Without question*, I tell myself as I stand above the toilet, *definitely, absolutely, if this is bloody again, then I will go to the campus infirmary.*

Bloody it is. More blood than anything. It's as if I'd swallowed red food coloring by mistake, as if the whole thing was some elaborate practical joke. There is no pain. It does not sting or burn. But blood pours out of my body in a way that it should not.

I stalk back to my room and pull on a pair of sweatpants. Most of my clothes are dirty. Rooting through the pile on the bottom of my closet, I find a reasonably clean sweatshirt. No time to take a shower first (*at least there's some sense of urgency, now*) but I do still brush my teeth, spitting more blood into the sink. I slip bare feet into my well-worn Keds and storm outside.

The walk across campus is a lonely one. The infirmary is at the far north end of campus, well past the end of the Spine. On weekends, Lancaster University gets fairly deserted. Many students go home. There are only a few people up and about this morning, mostly around the library, and even fewer after I branch off north toward the outskirts of the campus. The wind has picked up again, blowing hard from the northwest. It tears across the top of the hill. It cuts through my thin denim jacket. My sweatshirt isn't doing much to keep me warm. Rain-soaked grass numbs my feet when I try to take a shortcut. I am cold and wet and frightened. I am not prepared.

A sign on the outer door of the infirmary says that they are closed on weekends: *In case of emergency, please ring the bell. There will be a sister on duty.* I hesitate for a moment, debating whether or not this can wait two more days. The image of a twice-bloodied toilet bowl convinces me to stay. I ring the bell a few times before the door finally makes a series of unlocking sounds. A short woman pulls it open. She smiles and invites me inside.

"How can I help you?" she asks.

I'm thinking about how best to summarize the past couple of weeks. I don't have a chance to say anything before she speaks again.

"One second," she says, moving behind me to close the door. "Let us talk where it's warmer."

She leads me through the dark and empty waiting room to an expansive, high-ceilinged examining room. There are charts on the walls. Two low tables jut out into the center of the room, crisp paper stretched across the tops. Counters line the walls. At the far end of the room is a good-sized wooden desk. It is bathed in a soft light from the tall window behind it. Cotton swabs, Kleenex boxes, tongue depressors, and several loose manila folders decorate the desk. The sister sits in a brown leather chair.

"Now, then." she says, picking up a small pad of paper before looking up at me. "What can I do for you?"

I start to explain some of my general symptoms. Just a few things, off the top of my head: tired, feverish, sick and tired for days.

"More than anything else," I tell her, "it has been this intense fatigue. I just can't shake it. But there are other things. A bunch of bruises. And see these?" I say, lifting my upper lip. "A bunch of sores. I don't know why."

She removes a tongue depressor from a bluish jar. "Hmm," she says.

"And I guess the really important one happened earlier this morning. It's why I'm here. My urine was all bloody."

"Bloody? Was it painful? Did it burn?"

"No. It wasn't — it didn't. But it really freaked me out!"

She nods her head. "Yes, yes. Well, I'm certainly glad you came in. Do you think I could get a urine sample?"

"I'm not sure. Maybe. I've already gone twice this morning."

She gives me a glass of water to drink, and a plastic cup to pee in. "The bathroom is just over there," she says. "Take your time. Please try."

There isn't much to the sample, but what little I was able to force out is once again completely red. The sister rubs her right eyebrow with two fingers.

"Right," she says, deep in thought. "The fevers and such I can understand. There has been a bug going around, and I can understand that. I'd prescribe plenty of rest and Vitamin C…"

She pronounces it *vit-uh-men*, which is one thing I've come to love about living in England.

"But those sores on your mouth. The bruises you'd mentioned. And this bloody urine. I am afraid there's something more at work, here, something beyond my understanding. I am going to ring the doctor on call. He lives just a few minutes away. I hope I can reach him. He should have a much better idea of what's going on."

She steps away from the desk to make the phone call in another room. I'm too tired to think. When she returns, she relaxes in her brown leather chair, hands folded carefully in her lap. She asks me if I've been enjoying my stay in Lancaster. How long have I been here? Where am I from in the States? What classes have I been taking? Where are some of the places I've been able to visit? Scotland? Ireland? Europe? We talk for ten or fifteen minutes without saying a word about my health.

The doctor comes blustering in from the cold. His cheeks are red. He smiles and shakes my hand. His gloveless hand is cold against mine. The sister stands up and offers him her chair; he shakes his head no, then leans up against the edge of the desk closest to me. He is maybe forty-five, fifty, with a salt and pepper beard. His eyes are dark and questioning. More of the same questions as before, with more of the same answers. He uses a cotton swab to dab at the numerous sores inside my mouth. He shines a pocket light into my eyes, then down my throat.

"Tell you what," he says, after only a cursory examination. "I have a colleague at the Royal Lancaster Infirmary. It's right in town here. My friend — Dr. Lorigan — well, I'd like for him to take a look at you as soon as possible."

"But I don't have a car or anything. I'm not sure how I'd get there."

"Not to worry," he says, chuckling. "The sister here will drive you. We'd spoken about this possibility when she rang me earlier. I'll stay here. There are some details I'll want to share with Dr. Lorigan before you arrive. I'd expect he'll want you to spend the night, what with the way you've been bleeding. You should stop by your room to gather a few things first."

"What do you think is wrong?" I ask.

His smile is warm and comforting. "Too early to say. I'll let my colleague sort that out for you. Not to worry. You'll be in very good hands."

"Do you think I'll be there long? I mean, should I tell anybody?"

"Too early to say. Plan on staying at least the night, as I'd said, but beyond that I can't really say."

He reaches out to shake my hand again.

"Good luck to you, son."

CHAPTER 4

Things move quickly now. The sister walks with me to her Peugeot that's parked on the ring road behind the infirmary. It has clean front seats. We drive to one of many empty parking spaces adjacent to Pendle, not far from my open window. I throw a few odds and ends into my backpack: some reading from my Shakespeare and Victorian Lit classes, notebooks, my Walkman, a few mix tapes, extra batteries, deodorant, my shower kit. I'm not sure what else I need. I don't even know if I need these things. Can't keep standing around, though. Need to get moving.

I'd closed and locked the window behind me, after I'd crawled through it. Now with a heavier than usual backpack slung over one shoulder, I close and lock my door on the way out. I bump into Wayne in the hallway, briefly, stopping just long enough to share the condensed version of my day: woke up pissing blood, am getting a lift to the hospital in town to meet with some doctors. I'll be there for at least the one night. Maybe longer. I don't know anything else yet, but I promise to call him with more details later.

It's not long after that and the sister is guiding me through Royal Lancaster Infirmary. It is old and worn and feels massive. It feels like a maze. We wind our way through claustrophobic corridors. Paint flakes from the walls and ceiling. We stop outside a small room, where we are greeted by a stocky man wearing a white coat.

"You must be Robert," he says, shaking my hand briskly. "I'm Dr. Lorigan. Very pleased to meet you. So glad you're here."

He reminds me of the first doctor, the one from the campus infirmary, except he's maybe a little bit younger, and doesn't have any sort of beard. Maybe it's the eyes. He looks at me with a mix of confidence and concern.

"This is for you," he says, gesturing to a room on my left.

It is immediately across the hall from what looks to be some kind of nurse's station — I mean "sister's station," which is what nurses are called here (at least all the ones I've met so far). There is a large, wide window that looks into my room from the hallway. Opposite that is a much smaller window, square, that looks out to what appears to be an alley, a narrow open space between brick exterior hospital walls. A simple bed rests in the middle of the room, covered with crisp white sheets and a thin white blanket. There is barely enough space to walk along either side of the bed. The room is sparse and efficient. It surprises me that I have my own room. There is a vast ward ahead and to the right, past the sister's station, with dozens of beds lined up no more than five feet away from each other, light curtains separating them. But here I have my own bed, and walls, windows, a door. Why so much privacy? Perhaps because I'm an exchange student?

"This is mine?" I ask, a little uncertain about the arrangement. It can't be more than a few hours after I'd first walked up to the campus infirmary. My mind is moving slowly, like slogging through mud, constantly trying to catch up with new information. And what with all this walking and driving and handshakes and new faces, I'm just barely getting by on my twelve or thirteen hours of sleep from the night before. I haven't forgotten about fatigue, exactly, but the sight of that bed, and the promise that it's mine, brings it back to the front of my consciousness.

"You might as well make yourself comfortable," Dr. Lorigan says. He pats the bed.

"What's next?" I ask. "Do I have to do anything?" I'm thinking a nap would be nice. I'm hoping there's not much for me to do other than sleep, get some medicine, maybe get some food later. It occurs to me that I haven't eaten all day. Is that even allowed? Will they bring me food? Hospitals do that sort of thing, don't they?

"We're going to want a sample of your blood, first. A good sample. One of the sisters will be here in half a moment to help. She'll draw the blood. From there, depending on what the blood test tells us, we might want you to meet a specialist, here, a hematologist. He's fantastic. Dr. Gorst. Marvelous."

"A *what?*" I ask.

"He's a specialist," Dr. Lorigan says again. "A blood specialist."

He moves through the room, adjusting the blinds, checking the bed, lining up a row of empty plastic bottles on a small table underneath the large window next to my bed.

"We suspect something might have gone bad in your blood. This quick test, from the blood draw, this will help us understand more about what's happening. Dr. Gorst, he'll have some additional tests he might want to run, when he arrives later."

Dr. Lorigan stops short, as if remembering something.

"But I'm getting ahead of myself. What's next? Try to get some rest. We'll be just outside if you need anything."

"Thank you," I say.

The sister from the University, who has been standing in the hall, reaches through the door and hands me my backpack. She smiles tightly.

"Good luck to you," she says. I don't think she ever told me her name.

* * *

There's a small piece of gauze on the inside of my left elbow, held down by a thin strip of medical tape. The gauze has collected a good-sized circle of blood, seeping slowly outward, after the first of what I'm sure will be many needles poking into my arms to test this or analyze that.

Not long after the initial flurry of activity in my room — timed, I think, to make sure I'd fallen asleep for a quick nap — Dr. Lorigan is back to share the results of the earlier blood draws. He's all apologies, all polite and British and so, so very, very sorry about the news he needs to share: the results are not good. I want to make sure I understand. I've seen in movies where they say things like "the test results are negative" and everybody cheers because in medical movie terms, negative is positive. It's good to not have something bad. I ask for clarification, which he dutifully provides.

"Not good" is not the same thing as "negative," so when he says the results aren't good, he means just that. But he then quickly provides a "these tests are also not conclusive" caveat.

He knows, already, that my blood has gone bad. Of that there can be absolutely no doubt. It should be obvious to me, too, given all of the bruises and bleeding and whatnot, my own inconclusive and highly scientific "punch-my-leg-to-see-if-it-will-bruise test" notwithstanding. What we don't know yet is why. What's the root cause? What made my blood "go bad" in the first place?

That's why Dr. Gorst is on his way. Dr. Lorigan had paged him at home, earlier, almost immediately after I'd arrived, and told him a little about my situation. He doesn't normally work on Saturdays, or at least not this Saturday, so Dr. Lorigan had asked him to stop by to take a look and to potentially administer another type of test. Something to do with my bone marrow?

"This test will help eliminate uncertainty," Dr. Lorigan says. "It is important for us to know for certain what we're working with here, Robert. You'll like Dr. Gorst, I'm sure. He should be here before long."

* * *

Hours pass. The light outside has long since given way to the darkness of yet another cold and wet February night. I'm picking my way through a not-too-terrible dinner of baked chicken, potatoes, and Jell-O when there's a knock on my door.

An elderly man enters, carefully, gently. His white coat hangs loosely over a light, thin frame. A collection of pens stick out of the top of his breast pocket. Silvery-white hair thins out over the back of his head. He's flipping through several multi-colored pages on a clipboard as he walks closer to my bed, reading, smiling, nodding a brief acknowledgment to me.

"Dr. Gorst?" I ask.

"Yes," he says. "You must be Robert."

A male nurse enters the room after Dr. Gorst, pushing a metal cart. It jangles with equipment. Dr. Gorst looks around for a place for his clipboard, finally setting it on the edge of the metal cart. He lowers himself to the edge of my bed, hands on his thighs, a deep exhale as he sits down. He pats my legs underneath the blanket. It's easy enough to picture him as the kindly old country doctor, working in a rustic village, cobblestone streets and pubs that are as old as the churches (and centuries older than anything in America). It's a pleasant, glowing scene: Dr. Gorst casually strolling through town, smiling and waving at infants and retirees, all of them his patients at one time or another, he of the firm handshake and the always helpful advice. It's perfectly pastoral.

But then he's snapping green rubber gloves over his hands, asking, politely, if he can take a look at me, when there's really no question involved at all. I remember that he's here, in my private hospital room, because he's a hematologist. I don't even know what that means, not yet at least, but I figure that anything with an "ologist" at the end must be serious. There won't be any lollipops or smiley-face stickers for me after this visit.

Dr. Gorst asks to see the sores inside my mouth. He presses his fingers on either side of my neck when I say "ahh." He taps my back a few times while asking me to breathe normally. There's a stethoscope, probably, and lights, and notes taken by the male nurse standing nearby.

"Have you been bruising at all?" Dr. Gorst asks.

"A little," I tell him, taking my feet out from underneath the blankets. "There are a few bruises on the sides of my feet, there. See?"

"Yes. And these spots, too? What about these?" He points to a rash of tiny red dots, like pin pricks, running from the top of my feet up to my shins. I'd noticed them a couple of weeks ago. They don't itch. I tell him that I don't know what those are.

"Petechiae," he says.

"I'm sorry. What?"

"*Petechiae,*" Dr. Gorst enunciates. He looks more closely at both feet, lifting one ankle and then the other. "These spots, here, are called petechiae. It's blood, just underneath your skin.

"Would you mind turning over for a bit, son?" he asks.

I roll onto my stomach. He touches a few spots on my legs.

"You look like a punching bag back here," he says. I glance over my shoulder and see several purple and black bruises on the backs of both thighs.

"You can turn back over, now."

He waits quietly, patiently, as I prop myself back up against my pillows. He appears to be deep in thought, scanning through the sheets on the clipboard again.

"Well, then. That ices it." He nods to the male nurse. There's a green towel of sorts on top of the metal cart. Lifting first one corner, then another, the male nurse exposes a number of different needles. He starts working a pair of plastic gloves over his hands, too.

Dr. Gorst turns to face me again. I do my best to maintain eye contact.

"Do you know what a bone marrow aspiration is, son?"

"No. No idea. Some kind of a test? Testing my bones for something?"

He clears his throat. He turns to the male nurse. "Can I see that one... no... over there... yes. That's the one." The nurse hands him a long needle. It's easily a good six inches long. Thick. More like a knitting needle than something I'd expect to see in a hospital. He brings the needle closer, so I can see it.

"Yes, Robert. It's how we get what we need to test. This needle, here, is hollow. There is a little hollow tip at the end. Can you see it? We need to put this into your back, just above your tail bone, and retrieve a sample of your bone marrow. That's what we are after, really, your marrow. That's what we want to test."

"Okay," I say. "Is there anesthetic or anything? Are you going to have to put me under?"

"No. It might hurt a bit, but no. You'll be awake. It won't take long. We are going to have some anesthesia back there, just local, which will help. But I'll be honest with you: I'm going to need to put a good deal of pressure on your back. We need to push this through bone, understand? So it might take some work. You *will* feel this."

I nod.

"Good. Excellent. We'll go ahead and start now, if you'd just lie on your side. That way. On your left side. *Left.* Good."

I ask him if it would be easier if I removed my shirt. He tells me that would be fine, so I take it off then lay on my side. I'm looking through my small exterior window, trying to find something else to focus on. There's nothing to see. Metal clatters against metal behind me. Dr. Gorst clears his throat again. He whispers to the male nurse, and then I feel something cold on my lower back.

"Just cleaning the site, now, Robert." He dabs my back a few more times. "There will be a little poke here, now. This is the local anesthesia. It will be like a bee sting, and then I'll spread it around and things will start getting numb."

He shows me a much smaller needle. I appreciate the play-by-play. Really. I'm not sure what to expect, what to focus on, what to think, where to look, so I just try to breathe easy. And then the sting comes, exactly as he said it would. It is near my hip, on the right side of my back, the "up" side. My skin becomes tingly and numb. I can feel him working the needle around, spreading the anesthesia. He pushes against the skin. His thumb is there but I can't really tell anymore. The male nurse hands him a different needle. He pushes in more anesthesia. This time I don't even feel the second sting.

"You're doing fine, Robert. Just fine. I'm going to put the other needle in, now, the hollow one. Here is where you'll start to feel some pressure. You let me know if it hurts. If it hurts, you'll need to just let me know, and we can see about getting you more anesthesia. But you have to let me know, okay?"

My jaw tightens. *Breathe easy. Relax.*

I don't feel the needle enter my skin, but there is instant, steady pressure against my tail bone. Dr. Gorst grasps my hip with one hand. The pressure increases. Steadily. It doesn't hurt, not yet, not really, but I want to squirm away from it. I just want it to stop.

Before I know it, it's gotten much, much worse. *What the fuck?* What the hell is he doing back there? I'm trying not to picture what's happening, but what else can I do? I'm not doing a good job of imagining rainbows and unicorns and happy green meadows. My eyes are clamped shut, my jaws are tight, my stupid fucking logical brain trying to calculate how much force is required to puncture bone. I'm trying my best not to squirm away from the intense pain in my lower back.

The pressure subsides. Dr. Gorst releases his grip.

"You've got some good, strong bones there, son," Dr. Gorst chuckles. "How are you doing? Are you doing okay?"

I lick my suddenly dry lips. My voice cracks "okay."

"Good. Now, let's try again."

It's like he's trying to drive a fucking railroad spike through my spine. Didn't he get enough the first time? Did he even get the needle through? I can't imagine it getting any worse, but it does. The pain goes to eleven.

It does not occur to me to ask Dr. Gorst to stop. He'd told me to tell him when it got too bad, didn't he? But I know this isn't something you can anesthetize. I mean, I still can't actually *feel* the needle — it's just this steady, unrelenting pressure that's damn near unbearable. But that's not the needle. That's just force. I'm fighting with my body. I'm bearing down on every muscle, holding tight, trying to relax at the same time I'm trying to do whatever I can to keep myself from squirming away from Dr. Gorst's needle.

"There," he says, finally, sliding it out of my back. "That should be plenty." Somewhere behind me there is the sound of paper tearing. A dry cloth wiping at my back and then some kind of adhesive. There is a thick bandage. The pain is less sharp, now, but my back still hurts. I blink more tears away, then rub my face into the pillow.

Dr. Gorst stands up to leave while the male nurse collects equipment.

"You did quite well, Robert. Thank you. We should have results back for you within a few hours. At least the preliminary results. We'll need to run quite a few different tests, but I won't need to do another aspiration for those."

"Okay," I say. "Good. Thank you."

He chuckles. He's the old country doctor of my imagination again. Crow's feet at the corner of his smiling eyes, a lifetime of healing.

"I'm sure that hurt like the dickens, son, but you did just fine. More than fine. But now, I want you to get some rest. Sleep. That's the best thing for you now. We'll have the results for you by tomorrow morning at the latest."

CHAPTER 5

S unday is difficult, for more than a few reasons. The doctors have already told me, after my bone marrow aspirate last night, that I have "a bone disease." Dr. Lorigan and another doctor, a woman, woke me early in the morning. She tells me that they have narrowed it down. Dr. Lorigan tells me that it's in my bones. Then they both describe additional tests that are being run, additional work that Dr. Gorst will be doing to get a better picture of where we stand.

"We'll know more later," they promise. This is all the information I have, even without the detailed results of the bone marrow aspirate, the things about my body that I know for certain: extreme fatigue for the past week, if not more; bruises damn near everywhere (hands, back, legs, feet); tiny red dots speckled underneath the skin on my feet and shins; bleeding gums; sores all across the inside of my mouth (on my tongue, even); bloody urine; Dr. Lorigan's pronouncement that my "blood has gone bad;" and, most recently, the confirmation from my growing team of doctors that I have "a bone disease."

I hate listing things out like this. It sounds so much worse to me now. And as much as I'd like to delay what I have to do next,

I really can't. Not anymore. I may not have all the answers yet, but my family needs to know where I am. They need to have the same amount of mostly useless information that I do.

I buzz one of the sisters to ask if there's a phone I can use. None of the doctors or sisters want me to leave my room for any reason. They've even set up a portable toilet in one corner of the room, to go along with the plastic bottles used for collecting (and testing) my bloody urine. Just about a day into this and I understand that this room isn't for privacy, but for my protection.

Sara — a thirty-something sister, Scottish, amiable, with blondish brown hair pulled into a precise bun — wheels a rotary phone in on a wooden cart. A long cord dribbles out underneath my door, across the corridor to the office. I had planned on calling much later. Past eleven o'clock at night, again, for the cheaper long-distance rates. But I'm in the hospital. *Bone disease.* If this doesn't qualify as an emergency, I don't know what does, expensive overseas phone bills be damned.

The phone rings once. Twice. Mom picks up before the third ring.

"Robert! I'm so glad you called!" She is jubilant. "I was expecting your call — Laura told me you'd tried to call earlier in the week — but I won't be here this afternoon, so I would have missed you. I was hoping you'd call again today. And you did!"

"Why would you have missed me?" I ask. Delay tactics. "Where are you going?"

"To the theater," she says. She is happy, talking fast. It is morning back home in Seattle. I imagine her pacing with the phone, moving from the kitchen through the dining room, to the living room and back. She cradles the phone under her neck and talks with her hands. "We're all going to the Fifth Avenue, Donna, Janet, everybody. We're all meeting for lunch downtown, then maybe some shopping — Nordstrom's is having a sale — and then we're going to see... what was the name of it ... I have the tickets here. Oh, yes. *The Unsinkable Molly Brown*. It's supposed to be quite good."

"Sounds like a great time," I say.

"It should be. You know I always enjoying going out with the girls." Small talk. The knowledge, in the back of my mind, that have to come out and say it. I have to make the leap. My heart thumps. I do not know how to bring up this topic. There is a pause in the conversation, and I know I need to take it. My mother has to know. She starts to tell me more about her plans for the day, but I interrupt her.

"Mom, I have some bad news. Some pretty bad news, I think, but we're still not entirely sure."

There's a depth of silence. Probably only a beat or two but it feels much longer. I can imagine my mother's jaw tightening against the phone, her body suddenly tense. Shoulders, arms, everything. She's not pacing anymore. Her eyes stare at a point on the wall. They do not focus on anything in particular. Suddenly, the only thing that exists in her world is the tenuous phone line between us.

"What's wrong?" she asks.

"I'm in the hospital. In Lancaster. I've been pretty sick. The doctors say that they aren't sure yet. They want to run some more tests. We've done a few already. They're pretty sure that I have a 'bone disease.' That's what they told me this morning, at least. Something in my bones is making my blood go bad."

I try to describe my symptoms from the past week, the events from yesterday. She is crying, now, and it is difficult to know if she hears me. Does she know something I don't? I'm not sure what to say, so I keep telling her that it will be okay, that the doctors say I will be fine.

"It'll be okay, Mom..."

She starts peppering me for facts. "When did you do this? Where are you? What are the names of these doctors, where are you, what is happening? What do you mean by bone disease?"

And then she cannot speak. She sobs into the phone. I can't understand what she is saying. There is a heavy clunk from across the Atlantic. Paul, my stepdad, comes on the line. I ask him how the Sonics are doing. He asks what my mom is so upset about, did I flunk out of school or something? *Ha-ha!* I tell him that I am in the hospital. Nothing serious, maybe, just the hospital in Lancaster because I've been sick lately, might probably be a bone disease but Mom thinks it is worse than it is. You know how she can get sometimes. A wink and a nod.

"Hold on," he says. "Your mother wants to talk to you again."

She starts talking immediately. Composed. She has a pad and pen with her. She is precise, in control.

"Give me the names of your doctors. Last names are fine. What is the name of the hospital again? The Royal Lancaster Infirmary? How long have you been there? What *exactly* did they tell you? Are you on any medications? What is the time zone thing again?"

There is no tone or pitch to her voice. I answer her questions as best I can. She is struggling to hold back the flood waters. She asks me what they think it is and I tell her what I've been hearing from Dr. Gorst and others, about bad blood, about bone marrow, about uncertainty. And then she is wailing again.

"Hold on," she says, "Just hold on. I'm going to get your sister." She brings the phone down the hall and pounds on Laura's door. The sounds are muffled. There are a few more indistinct sounds and then my sister is on the line.

I already know what I am going to say to Laura. I have known for the better part of the day. I'd actually *rehearsed* it, surprisingly. It was earlier, after all the doctors had left, when I knew that I was going to have to call home. You have to understand that I dreaded making this call like no other phone call in my life. I'm in a small room in a small hospital in Lancaster, England. The room faces a narrow, brick-walled alley. There is an IV running into my arm. Two bags, one yellow, one clear, drip slowly into a tube that runs into my right arm. I can't even leave the room to go to the bathroom. My urine, being collected in bottles, is still more blood than anything. I am having difficulty understanding the situation myself; how am I supposed to explain it to my family?

Laura and I are close. We are much closer now than we were in high school, or grade school. When we were younger, sometimes, we would come home and fight. More than just words. We would punch and scratch. There would be bruises. Siblings fight. That's what we did. Even with that, though, we'd look out for one another. Especially Laura, looking out for me. Protective.

There was a kid named Jeff who lived across the street from us. He was a year older than me, a year younger than Laura. Jeff and I had built a tree house in third or fourth grade. It was in the low maple next to his driveway. The tree house wasn't all that high, no more than six feet above ground, nestled in thick, forking branches. We'd formed a secret club, away from mothers and sisters. I'm not even sure how it happened, but one day he threw me out of the club. Literally. The ground was hard, shitty splotches of dead grass. I'd landed on my back. He jumped down next to me. Then he pounced, sitting on top of me, tapping my chest with his fingers. He weighed more than me and I couldn't move. It was driving me crazy. He tapped and tapped and pretended that he was going to spit in my face.

And then Laura came out of nowhere, a flying tackle that sent Jeff sprawling. She hit him. We'd had enough practice fighting with each other that she'd gotten pretty good at throwing punches. But she also knew that this wasn't her little brother that she was beating on; the rules were a little different. She tore at his hair. He screamed. He tried to get away but she had him pinned. Laura told him that if he ever tried to hurt me again then she'd be back for more.

Now she's on the phone, not even half awake, asking me what is happening. "What's wrong with Mom?" she asks. "What did you do?"

"Laura," I say. "I really fucked up this time."

Please be on my side. Protect me. I am your baby brother and I need you to take care of me.

❋ ❋ ❋

I give myself a few minutes before calling Dad and Jane. I know that this will be the much easier phone call, having already broken the news to family once, but I still need some time to collect my thoughts.

Maybe ten years ago or so, give or take, Laura and I went on a camping trip to Montana with Dad and Jane. We had lots of great summer vacations with them growing up: fishing for rainbow trout at Yellowstone, a memorable hike with our Uncle Tom, too, in the Wind River mountain range on the edges of Wyoming and Montana.

This one year, though, when I couldn't have been much more than ten, we'd visited Flathead Lake, a little north of Missoula. One of Jane's college roommates had a cabin there and had invited all the extended families out for a week. We'd driven from Seattle, taking I-90 most of the way. Laura and I piled into the back of Dad's old Ford Courier pickup truck, sandwiched between sleeping bags, backpacks, fishing poles, tackle boxes, a couple of coolers. We read and slept and squabbled almost the entire way there.

But once we'd arrived? Oh, the pristine lake. The cabin tucked into the woods, just up the hill from twin docks. The promise of an afternoon spent water-skiing underneath the lazy summer sun, so hot it hums.

All the kids — probably half a dozen of us, Laura and I older than most — congregated on the front porch of the cabin. None of us were able to contain the energy that had built up over days of road-tripping to Montana from all points on the compass. We buzzed with ideas. The lake beckoned. One of the oldest boys, about Laura's age, suddenly yelled out "race to the docks!"

And we bolted, scampering off the porch, kicking up dust from the gravel road back down the hill to the lake. The bright glimmer of sunlight off the water caught my eyes. A shortcut appeared between the dense growth of pine and fir and juniper trees. The other kids took the zig and the zag of the long gravel driveway, winding slowly toward the shore, but I was smart. I was a clever little boy, ducking and weaving my way off the beaten path. I'd taken the far more direct route. I had the upper hand.

Here's something I've learned about forestry over the years: when trees grow next to steep drop-offs, roots will sometimes become exposed. A clever boy, with his eyes focused on the wide stretch of brilliant blue water on the horizon, might miss such things. He'd probably be running so fast that a barely noticeable group of roots that had formed a kind of hook between the tree and the ground would be enough to trip him up.

I flew into the air. The ground dropped away beneath me. It felt like I was miles into the Montana sky. As I quickly dropped down the few feet of rough, steep hill that ran parallel to the gravel road, I was able to at least get my feet underneath me. I tried to keep running but it was no use. I had no balance. I planted one foot down, and maybe got the second one underneath me before I ended up sprawled across the road. Tiny pebbles embedded themselves in my hands as I slid to a stop. Skin peeled away from both knees and elbows. Dirt and dust surrounded me. My cries shattered the calm of an otherwise perfect afternoon.

That shocking, stupid, instantaneous pain wasn't nearly as bad as what came later, after Laura had helped me back up to the cabin. There were tweezers and peroxide and expectations when Jane worked to extract the various bits of rock and dirt from my skin. I sat on the edge of a kitchen counter, trying to keep my legs still, biting down on a rough white towel to keep from crying out again.

The setting sun burned off the lake, casting long shadows through the dining room windows. That's where I wanted to be — on the white boat I couldn't see behind me, speeding through the water, holding on desperately to an inner tube as we bounced across the wake.

This is what I'm thinking about when I call Dad and Jane. This is the story that I lead with when Dad answers the phone. Jane picks up the second handset so I can talk with them at the same time. They're both anxious, and worried, and try to get to some of the same answers through some of the same questions. It's the same stunned disbelief. It's barely been a few months since they'd seen me over the Christmas Holiday. How can I be in the hospital? How did this happen? How?

Already I'm trying to make light of everything, already trying to put everyone's mind at ease. *It's not so bad*, I tell them, over and over, *it's nothing to worry about.*

CHAPTER 6

There's a knock on my door. It's late in the afternoon, pushing into the evening. Expecting one of the doctors — hoping for official results from Dr. Gorst, even though Sara had mentioned that it might not be until tomorrow, now, before we know — I'm surprised, instead, to see Simon, and Wayne. They're both wearing surgical masks. After the first tentative knock, they spill boisterously into my room.

I'm lucky to have had the opportunity to even meet these two, let alone appreciate how much I've come to value their friendship these past months. Wayne's room is directly across mine at Pendle. Simon is down the hall, his room facing the interior courtyard like Wayne's. They'd immediately welcomed me into their group of friends, my bland American accent notwithstanding.

That I've been an American student living in an English dorm (or "college") is the result of a conscious choice I'd made some time ago. Carleton College gives students ample opportunities to study abroad, typically during their junior year. Most of those programs, including ones in London and Paris and even China, mean you travel to those countries with a Carleton professor and take classes with other Carleton students. While those are still great opportunities to travel and see the world, they'd always felt more like extended field trips to me than a true study abroad program.

That's what Lancaster is. I've actually transferred here for my fall and winter terms, an exchange student instead of a tourist. Living side-by-side with students from all over England, as well as another exchange student (David, from Paris, pronounced *Dah-veed*), was exactly what I'd wanted. I feel like I've been living here, not just visiting. That was important to me when I first started thinking about being able to spend my junior year overseas and is even more important now. These are my mates. They've got my back.

I'm smiling as I try to sit up in my bed a little.

"You never called yesterday," Wayne says. "So we got worried and came to find you. What's with the room? These masks?"

I try to catch them up on what I know, which frankly isn't much right now. I tell them about the bone marrow aspiration, and all the bleeding from yesterday and today, rolling over a bit to lift up the corner of my pajamas so that they can see the thick bandage.

"It's bad, yeah?" Simon asks. "They say your blood has gone bad? Your bones are doing that? So that means it must be serious, isn't it?"

"I think so," I say. "I should know more later today. But, yeah, I think it's serious. I probably won't be out in time to make it to any of my classes tomorrow."

Wayne tells me not to worry about my classes. "It's your pool match tomorrow night I'm worried about," he says. "We're going to have to scratch you from the team. I'm not sure who we'll get to fill in for you. If we bloody lose to Grizedale, it'll be your fault!"

Wayne and I laugh, but Simon doesn't join in. He looks like he's ready to ask me more questions that I won't know how to answer but is interrupted by another knock at the door. It's Sara, again. There have been a number of different doctors and sisters entering and exiting my room since yesterday, but it seems like we've settled into a kind of pattern. It's mostly Sara and Dr. Lorigan and Dr. Gorst now. Sara makes a beeline to my bed, checking first on the antibiotics I've been getting all day. She also wants to examine the site of the aspirate. Despite my best attempts to keep pressure on it — excluding the past handful of minutes — the bandage is soaked again.

Sara says that we need to change the bandage again. Plus, I need to eat some dinner that just arrived outside the door. And Dr. Lorigan has asked for another blood draw. With all of that, she says, it might be best if my visitors come back some other time. Maybe tomorrow, after I've had a chance to eat and rest. She gives them a long look.

After a quick hand on my shoulder and a "see you tomorrow," Wayne is out the door. Simon smiles weakly. He's reluctant to leave, but slowly follows after Wayne anyway. He pauses at the door.

"Seriously, mate" he says. "I'm here if you need anything. Anything at all. Just give us a ring, yeah?"

✳ ✳ ✳

It's night, I think. Late. My sense of time is starting to get shaky. It's dark outside and light inside and that doesn't help me one bit.

I wish I had a watch. I'm trying to piece together the last remnants of a dream — something about a chase, I was running after something, maybe, at the same time I was running *from* something? — when I realize that my tee-shirt and pajama bottoms are soaked through.

This has been happening the past couple of nights, waking up from feverish dreams and my clothes and sheets are damp with sweat. I didn't pack anything else to wear, though. I'm not sure what to do, and so I decide to roll over on my other side and see if I can fall asleep again, sweaty clothes and all.

That's when I realize that I haven't been sweating. This is blood. My right arm is a bloody mess. The IV that had been there is missing, pulled out who knows how long ago while I was thrashing my way through my dreams, and whatever vein it had tapped into must have kept pumping away. In the half light of my room I can see that my bed sheets are dark and damp, too.

More embarrassed than frightened, I stand up and move to the large window that looks out over the sister's station across the hall. Dr. Lorigan had been adamant that I was absolutely *not* to leave my room under any circumstances, so I begin awkwardly waving, trying to get the attention of one of the sisters there, miming through the window that I've somehow accidentally pulled the IV needle from my arm.

I'm light-headed. I feel like I need to sit back down again. Somebody opens the door and helps me to one of the chairs on the far wall. She cleans off my arm, wraps it with layers of white gauze. People are in and out. Bloody sheets and blankets and pillow cases are exchanged for clean ones. Anonymous hands help me out of my clothes, and a series of damp sponges wipe the blood away from my sides and back. They replace the bloody bandage from my bone marrow aspiration.

I can't stop apologizing. *I'm so sorry. I'm so sorry for all this trouble.*

My apologies are acknowledged and then hushed away. A fresh set of hospital-issued pajamas appears from somewhere. After we're certain that all the blood has been cleaned off my body, I'm helped into the pajamas and then guided back to bed. Sleep quickly overtakes me, before I have a chance to think about all the blood I've been losing.

✳ ✳ ✳

Morning finally arrives. Bad dreams persist, but I'm so tired that I haven't been able to avoid them. A fresh new doctor appears at my bedside. He introduces himself, but it's in one ear and out the other.

"I've been going through your charts," he says. "I understand you had something of an accident last night?"

"I guess."

"Yes," he says, nodding. "Could I see your arm, please? The one where we'd had your IV?"

I sit up as best I can, leaning against the pillows. I extend my right arm to him.

"Here," I say.

He takes hold of my wrist with one hand before running a finger along my forearm, up to my elbow, as if he were tracing the veins just below my skin.

"Sounds like quite the scare last night," he says.

"I know. I'm really sorry. I didn't mean to."

He twists my arm slightly, and then runs his hand back down to my wrist. Using two fingers, he taps at the base of my wrist a few times.

"No, no. No need to apologize. We just don't want you losing any more blood. Now let's see about getting this IV back where it belongs."

He wipes away some dried blood from the base of my wrist using a cool alcohol swab, then dries my skin with gauze. Suddenly, there's a sharp pain where the gauze had been. I look down. I should know better by now that doctors usually clean my skin so they can stick something into it. He's inserted a small needle at the very base of my wrist, on the top of my arm, right where it bends. He then re-attaches the tube from my IV to the end of the needle.

"What?" I'm confused. *Why did he put the needle there?*

"Don't worry," he says, reaching for some adhesive tape. He tapes both the needle and a small amount of the IV tubing to my wrist and forearm. "There," he says. "That should do it."

I try moving my wrist. It's awkward and uncomfortable. If I bend my wrist even a little, I can feel the needle poking me. The only way to avoid pain of the IV needle — which doesn't seem like it should be something that hurts — is if I hold my wrist perfectly still, perfectly straight.

"Look," I tell him. "This is really uncomfortable. Can't you put it in my forearm or my elbow or someplace?"

He shakes his head.

"That's the point, now, isn't it? To make sure that it doesn't come out again."

* * *

I'm sleeping so much. My body is still so desperate for sleep that I find myself nodding off at every opportunity. Even the uncomfortable needle jabbing my wrist doesn't keep me awake for long. During the winter in Lancaster, the days would often be covered in darkness. The morning would progress from black to a dim cloud-covered light, then slowly back again to darkness. It's hard enough to keep track of daylight without being stuck inside the confines of my hospital room. I've already lost my sense of day and night, lost it in all of those shades of gray.

My days are a confusing mess of dreams and nightmares and waking memories. It's not a dream when Dr. Gorst quietly re-enters my room. He's floating, I think, or walking so softly and quietly to make sure not to wake me if I happen to be asleep. He has news for me, news that he is glad that I'm awake to hear. The door clicks closed behind him.

He is calm and reassuring. His voice is low. Steady. Comforting. He tells me that the bone marrow biopsy had given him the details he needed. He wasn't surprised by the results, he says, as much as he'd hoped it might be something else.

Dr. Gorst sits on the edge of my bed. He does not mince words.

"I'm very sorry, Robert. You have leukemia."

CHAPTER 7

I 'd first heard Kate Bush while spending countless hours in the Pendle College JCR. There was a jukebox up against one wall, near the windows that looked out into the courtyard. I'd drop a pound coin into the slot and pick out a handful of songs to keep us company while we played pool in the evenings. I'd pick The Stone Roses, Neneh Cherry, Soul II Soul, New Order, The Smiths, Squeeze, among others. But mixed in from somebody else's selections came this amazing and ethereal voice singing about This Woman's Work. I started playing that song obsessively. Loved it so much that I caught a bus into Lancaster on a wet and windy afternoon to buy the tape it came from, The Sensual World.

It was one of the few non-mixtapes I'd packed with me over winter break. Traveling from Lancaster to London to Paris, and then on a train, solo, through France and Italy and a ferry ride to Greece, I must have played that tape on a near-endless loop. I'd spent New Year's Eve in a tiny hotel room in Athens with a sliver of a view of the Parthenon, drinking cheap champagne, welcoming in 1990 with three other Americans and an Australian couple on holiday I'd met earlier in the day.

The next morning, I'd rushed off to catch a train to Mycenae, on my own, to look for the beehive tombs of Clytemnestra and Agamemnon, and the famed Lion Gate. Kate Bush once again kept me company. It's hard to understate what her music meant to me, all of twenty years old, winding my way south through Europe — through history — for the first time.

It doesn't matter that the intended meaning behind the song applies to something completely different than what I'm facing right now. I know exactly what I need to listen to after Dr. Gorst leaves me alone with my cancer. Her tape is already in my Walkman. I'm sitting on the edge of my bed, my back turned away from the long interior window, holding my Walkman loosely between my legs, pressing stop, rewind, play. Stop, rewind, play. Stop. Rewind. Play.

I don't know what to think. I don't know what to do. I'm stuck here in England and I'm scared about what's happening. Kate Bush with her haunting, beautiful voice helps me feel like I'm not entirely alone. Tears roll down my face, under my chin, down my neck. I don't bother to wipe them away.

* * *

For the most part, I need to lay as flat as possible. I'm trying to rest on a paperback book I've placed just underneath the small of my back to keep pressure on that stupid bone marrow aspiration site. The doctors keep putting holes in my body, and my blood keeps spilling out of them. Sara comes in regularly to replace the bandage. She checks my temperature, adjusts the drip on my antibiotics, makes a few notes on the clipboard at the end of my bed.

"Can I get you anything else?" she asks. "Something else to eat? A movie to watch? Another blanket?"

Sara knows. Everyone in that room immediately across the hall from me knows what's happening inside my body. They are being exceptionally polite and helpful.

"No, no," I shake my head. "No, thank you."

She leaves me alone with my thoughts again. With headphones over my ears once more, an uncomfortable needle in my wrist, and water at the edges of my eyes, I let my imagination carry me back home.

My fingers press against closed eyes — thumb to the right, forefinger to the left. Push out, then back in, pinching the bridge of my nose. Slide down. Wipe the moisture on the bed sheets. Lower the volume on my Walkman. *What do I own?* It is a simple matter. It's practical. I don't know what I don't know. I don't know survival rates, don't know treatments, don't know anything other than the fact that for the first time in my life there is the very real possibility that I'm going to die. Probability? And it's all in slow motion, and everybody is so fucking *polite* about *everything*. All please and thank you and how can I help, whispering quietly to me in this piece of shit hospital in a piece of shit corner of the planet that's about as far away from home as I can imagine. I don't know a damn thing about anything and I'm angry at myself for that.

My first comic-book inspired vision of what a bone marrow transplant might look like involves a full skeletal replacement, like they'll dip me in a vat of some oozing bubbling liquid somewhere while my mutant healing powers will help me survive as every bone in my body is replaced with adamantium. How can I expect to have a serious conversation about the healing process when my brain won't let me imagine the words "bone" and "transplant" without immediately picturing Wolverine?

After Sara has shooed everyone out of my room, and it's finally just me and my bleeding bandages and a handful of tapes I'd been listening to for the past six months, Kate Bush on heavy repeat, I start to think about what I have. It's a will, isn't it? That's what you're supposed to do in situations like this, right? I might not die, sure, but I've got to start thinking about what I'm going to leave behind when I'm dead.

My mix tapes — with sides titled *New Funk Dance Shit*, *Mellow Mix*, *Fuckin A!*, and *Bee-Yootiful!* — songs that had been mapped out for consistency and style and transitions between artists, tempo, variety, well, I wouldn't want them to just get tossed in the trash after I died. I wouldn't want them to be forgotten. Would my sister appreciate them most? Laura has good taste in music. But what about roomies at Carleton? Aaron and Brady and I would DJ parties together — they both have excellent taste in music, too, and might appreciate something like that to remember me by.

But then what about my books? My Nintendo? My leather jacket? My Lynda Barry denim jacket, hanging over the edge of chair in the corner, autographed at a writer's conference from my senior year in high school, all tattered and faded but still important? What happens to that? What about the undeveloped photos lined up in film canisters on my bookshelf back at Pendle? I don't even know if any of those photos are any good. Who takes care of those? Or is it best, when making out a will in your head, to first identify the people you want to give things to, and then the stuff? I've never done this before. I don't have any experience.

The last thing I want to be doing is figuring out all the worthless crap I've managed to accumulate over two decades, but I can't stop. I feel like this is a necessary step. What if I don't even *have* a tomorrow to figure it all out?

God. I'm so fucking tired. I cover my face with both hands, just for a second, and then I'm being gently nudged awake. It's too easy to drift off like that. Close my eyes for a moment and I'm gone.

Sara's here to check on my bandages again. She asks me to lift up my back, just a little. "It's okay," she says, after a moment or two. "You have more visitors. Do you want me to ask them to come back?"

I try to push myself up into a kind of sitting position. My headphones have fallen around my neck. Through the window to my right there are two familiar and friendly faces peering inside: Colin and Rosemary Lyas. Yes! Absolutely. They are most welcome.

Colin — tall, dark-haired, thoughtful, possessing that famed dry British wit — is the advisor for the half dozen Carleton students here at Lancaster this year. He's a philosophy professor at Lancaster, and, as he'd shared with the group of us over beers on one of our many weekend excursions (*Lake District, you'll forever be my favorite*) he's also spent a couple of years teaching at Carleton, too. So he's had some direct understanding of the academic environment we've all come from. I'd assume he maintains regular contact with the Office of Off-Campus Studies, too. Colin has been a great resource these past months, both him and his petite, whip smart wife, Rosemary. They'd welcomed us into their homes immediately and continued to make us feel like we were part of an extended family instead of simply being exchange students.

How did they know I was here? News of my situation has obviously traveled fast.

"We came just as soon as we found out," Colin says as he and Rosemary approach the side of my bed. She wants to give me a hug, I know, but I'm still flat on my back. It's awkward. Instead, she smooths down a corner of my blanket, then reaches out to gently brush my cheek. Her hand lingers, briefly. Colin gives my right leg a paternal pat, and they both look at me with such true concern and compassion that I have to look away.

That's one of the other things to know about Colin and Rosemary: they're two of the nicest damn people you'll ever meet. They both start apologizing to me, and then I'm telling them that there's no reason to be sorry, that it's not their fault what happened. If anything, I'm the one who should be apologizing to them for causing such a fuss.

I'll begin to figure this out on my own, before too long. "I'm sorry" has multiple meanings, depending on the context. Of course it does. It turns out that Colin and Rosemary aren't apologizing, they're simply trying to express their sorrow. That's what "we're sorry" means when spoken to somebody who was recently diagnosed with cancer.

"We also want you to know," Colin says, "that we're here to help with anything you need. Absolutely anything."

Rosemary continues the thought: "Your mother will be flying out soon, yes? I'm happy to meet her at the train station whenever she's scheduled to arrive."

"And logistics," Colin says. "I can facilitate communication between Lancaster and Carleton, as necessary. You'll have course work you need to finish up, too. I can coordinate with your professors on what you'll need from each of them to wrap up your credits."

"*Anything*," Rosemary smiles.

As we talk through more of the ways they want to help, it occurs to me how much planning and coordination needs to happen yet. So many details that need to be sorted out between my doctors and my parents and insurance companies and airlines and at least a couple of different schools and hospitals. There is much work to be done. And that's just to get me to a place where I can start treatment, whatever that ends up being. Much work to be done, indeed.

There's no time — or even a very good reason anymore — to try to even think about finishing the will I'd started before Colin and Rosemary arrived. I do *not* need a reason to continue to feel sorry for myself, to slip away into sleep imagining who will come to my funeral, what they'll be wearing, the quotes they'll read about me, how many boxes of Kleenex they'll go through. It's time to focus on getting better. That's the only thing that matters any more.

My room at the Royal Lancaster Infirmary is this smallish rectangle with little space for anything other than the bed, and everyone is even more adamant than ever that I'm not to leave the room under any conditions, at least not until we're ready to move me for good. As friends have visited since Sunday, a gentle, steady, ever-expanding wave of smiling, worried faces from the University, they've tended to congregate at the foot of my bed. There's really no other place for them to stand. I'm able to see them as they pass the window on my right, approaching the door, then knocking first to make sure not to disturb my rest.

I do my best to explain what the IV is for, what the tests have been, and what the test results mean for me. I'm optimistic. I want my friends to smile and laugh and not worry about what might happen. I tell them that there's nothing to worry about, that survival rates are exceptional.

We're able to laugh. They bring gifts and get-well cards and hugs. I'm tired and scared and I don't want to say goodbye. Simon reassures me that he'll do whatever he can to help out when Mom arrives.

It's strange: as the details of my departure are arranged behind the scenes, planned between my parents and doctors at multiple hospitals and insurance companies and airlines, I feel like I haven't really done anything since I got here. There's been all this motion, all these people coming and going, drugs and antibiotics and needles and bleeding, all these lists and phone calls and sleep-filled days. Friends say their goodbyes, some with laughs, others with tears. They leave my room, smiles and waves trailing along the window until they disappear beyond my field of vision. It feels like I'm not the one leaving Lancaster, but that my friends are the ones leaving me.

CHAPTER 8

I t's been clear, almost immediately after Dr. Gorst told me I had leukemia, that my treatment would begin somewhere else. London, maybe. The Royal Lancaster Infirmary simply isn't equipped. I would need to leave this hospital, this city, sometime in the very near future.

While I may not consistently be awake enough or aware enough to feel any concern, or to participate in any of the behind-the-scenes planning, there is still a constant sense of urgency surrounding me. I feel it all around me. A small thing, like the chart affixed to the end of my bed. There is information on that clipboard that I know nothing about. The sisters come into my room throughout the day, taking my temperature, my blood pressure, asking how I feel. Every so often they might withdraw more blood. Numbers and letters fill the charts. Dr. Lorigan reviews the numbers and letters. He confers with Dr. Gorst. They call my parents and share important details and discuss options and give direction to Sara and the other sisters who come into my room again, rousing me from my slumber, asking me to swallow this small plastic cup of thick medicine that tastes like bananas or that pill that makes me gag and retch.

So much activity, so much to worry about, so many plans being made all around me. About me, but not without me.

It's a rough sketch, at first, but the details slowly begin to fill in. London is crossed off the list. My treatment, whatever that will be (*but certainly not being dipped into a vat for a full skeletal replacement*) is going to be involved enough, and lengthy enough, that it makes the most sense for me to be back in The States to start it. Everybody is very matter-of-fact with me. These things make sense. It's clear, and logical, and there really aren't any other options.

A handful of facts that have become clear in the last day or so. First, I'd waited perhaps a bit too long before mustering the courage to visit the University Health Centre. Leukemia is fast. At least that's what they're telling me about my particular type, Acute Mylo-something Leukemia. AML. Because I'd waited so long, and because my blood so clearly keeps trying to leave my body when it shouldn't, I'm now something of a considerable travel risk. While everyone absolutely wants me to make it back across the Atlantic in one piece, there's some understandable concern from the airlines about my current health and liabilities and so forth.

Because of that risk, it has been mandated (whether by the Royal Lancaster Infirmary or the insurance company, I do not know) that I be joined in my travels by both a doctor and a nurse. Mom is already on her way here. The four of us will all be leaving Lancaster together not long after she arrives. We'll get to London somehow, then board a plane that will take me to a hospital. The doctor and nurse are from the Royal Air Force. They will make sure I get to my destination safely.

We will be flying non-stop. Period. There is no room for discussion about this. Not only will it be the fastest route, but it minimizes any additional danger moving me between aircraft. The flight will depart from London and land in either Minneapolis — if my treatment is going to be at the Mayo Clinic — or Seattle.

Turns out that I'm extremely lucky, all things considered. I get to go back home. Either option would have brought me to a place that feels like home, but only one of those is where all my family and childhood friends are located. Between the doctors and my parents and the insurance company, it's decided that my treatment will be at the University of Washington Medical Center.

It seems odd at first, but one of the final pieces of the plan requires the purchase of six airline seats just for me. There will be three other seats for my traveling companions. I'm not entirely sure why I get six seats all to myself, but maybe it's to make sure there's room for hooks to hang for any antibiotics or blood that might need to drip down during the flight home.

The cost of all of this boggles the mind. Six one-way tickets for me, and two round-trip tickets for the RAF doctor and nurse, all purchased only a few days from when we'll need to leave. Not to mention Mom's round-trip flight to come get me. It's already staggeringly expensive, and we haven't even started treatment yet!

* * *

Mom has always been afraid to fly. Used to be prohibitively petrified. A combination of claustrophobia and being out of control kept her away from both airplanes and elevators for much of my childhood. In the latter case, one could always find a set of stairs. In the rare instances that there weren't, or it meant too many steps, then the tense, nerve-wracking ride would at least be mercifully short. Not so for airplanes.

As Laura and I got older, there were places Mom wanted to go to that couldn't be easily reached by road or rail. She took a series of classes when I'd just started high school to help with her fear of flying. The graduation "ceremony" involved a short trip: Seattle to Portland and back. Even though she'd learned the principles behind lift — how something much heavier than air could remain suspended thousands of feet above ground — and she knew the different sounds one could expect during a flight, she sat through the ride to SeaTac airport for her first flight with a pale, sunken face. Her entire body was so rigid and tense during the drive that Laura and I didn't say a word. Laura was driving, giving Mom one less thing to worry about, and I sat quietly in the back, thinking that maybe even one word — one breath — and she'd tell Laura to turn the car around and drive us all back home.

We made it, though. She made it to the airport with only a few tears shed. A few of her close friends — Donna, Gail, and Janet — met us at her gate. They were able to joke with her, offer words of encouragement. This was her trip. It was great support, but she knew that she needed to do this all by herself. She needed to own it. When it came time to board, she looked back at us, her face hollow and horrified. One of the few times that I'd ever seen my mom truly, visibly *afraid*. When she'd returned the next day, she was still visibly stressed, but also light on her feet, a palpable weight lifted from her shoulders.

"Well," she'd smiled. "I did it!"

We still rarely took family vacations that required air travel, but at least she'd managed to conquer her fears.

And now in a matter of days, she's learned that her only son has leukemia; has managed to get a new passport, somehow, in less than 24 hours; is flying to England for the first time in her life; will take a several hour train trip from London to Lancaster; and then later tonight, she will accompany said sick child (*yours truly*) in an ambulance right back to where she'd arrived in England.

It'll be a whirlwind tour to say the least. Running on fumes and fear and parental concern, trusting that jet lag won't even have a chance to set in. It's safe to say that I'm expecting she will be a complete wreck when she arrives. Like I'm one to talk.

* * *

The hardest part, at first, is that I can see her through the window before she can actually come into my room. She's with Colin and Rosemary and one of her best friends, Gail who'd by chance been in London visiting her daughter and not only met Mom at Heathrow but took the train all the here with her, too. I'm guessing that Colin and Rosemary must have met them both at the Lancaster train station to ensure that they found their way to my hospital room.

I'd gotten up out of bed when I first saw the entourage in the hallway and have been trying to clean up a bit. It's embarrassing. I don't know what to do about all the bottles of my pinkish urine stacked on a low table next to the window, you know, so I just straighten them up. Like this is my bedroom or something, and it has to be tidy when Mom visits. My mouth tastes awful, so I brush my teeth quickly, too, once again spitting out bloody foam.

She's smiling and waving from the hallway and looks like she hasn't slept in days. She looks like she's been crying nearly all that time, too. And she can't come into my room until Dr. Lorigan is able to track down one of the sisters to find surgical masks for everyone. Obviously, we're trying to minimize physical contact, which has to be hard for Mom at the end of a long journey. She's crying again, when she's finally able to burst through the door.

There are hugs all around. Mom is first, longest, and last. I thank Colin and Rosemary for being here. Gail, too. That's three more people than I'd expected to see when Mom arrived. It's nice to see how quickly support networks can form. She's needed this, I know.

We talk about logistics. Blood transfusions, antibiotics, the ambulance scheduled to come at midnight tonight. She wants to know what to do about everything in my dorm room. She's concerned that there's not enough time to get everything before we need to leave.

I give her my room key. Tell her how to get to Pendle College, my room number, all of that. Rosemary assures her that they'll be able to drive her anywhere she needs to be. I also give her my ATM card and write the PIN down on a piece of notebook paper so she can withdraw everything. There's room to write down a few directions for stuff I'd still like to bring home: a few favorite tee-shirts, more books that I'll want, more tapes, just more clothes in general that I'm sure I'll need when I get to the hospital in Seattle.

"If you see anybody, Simon or Wayne or anybody, could you please tell them I'm sorry? Tell them I didn't mean to leave so suddenly."

Mom and Gail don't think it's very funny when I tell them about how we'd all been playing pool together, not that many days ago, and we were joking about cancer.

We don't have much time to visit. Colin and Rosemary invite both Mom and Gail back to their house after the quick stop at my dorm room.

"I have a wonderful Paella recipe I'd like to share with you," Rosemary says. She takes my mom's hand in hers. "And wine and cigarettes, too, if you want."

Mom quit smoking years ago, but I can see the sparkle in her eye. I thank Colin and Rosemary again. More hugs all around as they prepare to run a variety of errands on my behalf before returning late tonight. There's not much time left now.

* * *

Mom and Gail are at Colin's house getting some rest and a meal. Mom had called earlier to let me know that she'd be back here in a few hours, by about 10:30 or 11:00, plenty of time before the ambulance arrives. She'd told me Rosemary's paella was delicious. Colin had built a fire and the four of them have been enjoying a couple of bottles of wine together.

I'd suggested that she should try to take a nap. Has she slept at all since I'd called her? I doubt it. If so, it can't have been much. I'm lucky. Even when I start to worry about things, my body wants to help me drift off into sleep.

Except right now. I'm too nervous and excited. Everything changes now. This wasn't at all how I'd expected to be leaving

Lancaster, and I don't know that I'm ever coming back. I also don't have any idea what it's going to take to beat this disease.

I mean, I know it's cancer, and I know that lots of people do not survive it. But I'm also fairly certain that it's something that people survive all the time, too. It's an afterschool special sort of disease, right? I'll lose my hair and people will hover and worry, but I'll get through it. Easy.

It's quiet. My room hasn't been this empty and quiet all day. I dig around in my backpack for my journal. I thought I'd brought it with me, or asked Simon to bring it with him, but I can't seem to find it. No matter. There's some paper here I use for my classes. I pull the food tray up closer to my bed so I can have a hard surface to write on. I want to get some clarity before I leave Lancaster, maybe forever. I want to get my thoughts in order.

This is what I write:

28 Feb 1990

Some thoughts: people have been asking me one question over and over: how do you feel? They want to know how I'm dealing with the knowledge that I've got a malignant disease — a cancer — and that I very well could DIE from it, if not treated carefully. I don't know. I'm still shaping my opinions, but they basically boil down to one analogy.

It's as if a small boy squats down, in the summer, to look at a beetle walking by. With one casual tip of his forefinger, the boy flips the beetle onto its back.

He walks away, laughing. Perhaps he's going to get a magnifying glass. I don't know. The point is, what does the beetle do? Does he lay on his back, slowly blistering in the sun, thinking "Gee, that's not really fair," or "Damn it, why me, why not the next beetle? Why me?" or even "No. This isn't happening. This can't be happening."

You can be damn sure none of those thoughts enter his meager little brain. What he does is start kicking and rocking and flailing, doing everything in his power just to survive. To me, that's all that matters: getting well. I've got leukemia, and I'm certainly not happy about it, but I've got a future to think of.

There will be no crying over spilled milk, only a voice in the kitchen saying "could you toss me a rag, please? I've got a real mess to clean up."

✳ ✳ ✳

The ambulance is scheduled to arrive around midnight to take the four of us — Mom, myself, and both the nurse and the doctor from the Royal Air Force Medical Corps — to Heathrow. Our midnight departure from Lancaster is intentional. We're working backwards from when the flight is supposed to take off, sometime mid-morning tomorrow. This allows for several hours to get settled in at Heathrow, to go through whatever security and/or medical checks might be required. We're also leaving well in advance of that to ensure that we'll miss that mess on our way into London. The goal is a nice, quiet drive through the darkened English countryside. No sirens needed.

There will, however, be a blood transfusion for me. Transfusions, really, the first of many pints of blood I'll be receiving on the ride to London. The doctors also talked about giving me some platelets later this afternoon. I'd never even heard the word before, "platelets."

"It's the part of your blood that helps it clot," one of my had doctors explained. "You've been bleeding so much. Platelets, first, to help thicken things up a tad, so to speak. Then blood transfusions, later, while you're traveling in the ambulance, to make up for what you've lost."

I have lost *so* much blood recently: every time I go to the bathroom, still, from my gums, from puncture wounds on my back, after my stupid, senseless thrashing around in my sleep. A few pints of liquid refreshment (*real, honest, whole blood*) should give me some much-needed energy.

I imagine I'll feel a little like a vampire, being loaded into my ambulance under the cover of a dark and foggy night in England. There will be a treat for me there: a new bag filled with blood, a steady drip into my system to be enjoyed while I continue to rest. My doctor explains that I'll receive fresh bags of blood periodically — as many as three or four, depending on how long it takes us to get to London. And then we will take to the skies in the morning, the four of us racing after the sun.

CHAPTER 9

We leave Lancaster almost exactly on time. Precision. There are brief introductions, all around, between the ambulance drivers, the doctor and the nurse traveling with us, Mom, myself. Polite greetings. Stifled yawns. I'm so groggy. How did I manage to stay awake until midnight? Probably the forty-seven some naps I'd taken throughout the day leading up to our departure.

Dr. Lorigan has stayed late to ensure a smooth hand-off to the Royal Air Force doctor and nurse. In addition to the new infusion of blood, I continue to receive a steady diet of antibiotics. We double-check that all my charts are in order, that blood and antibiotics are flowing down clear plastic tubes, letting gravity do the work all the way into my right arm.

Mom pushes me through the hallways of the Royal Lancaster Infirmary in a wheelchair, slowly, cautiously, taking extra care. Dr. Lorigan walks next to us. An orderly carries my backpack and a small bag containing a few miscellaneous things that Mom and Gail had picked up from my room earlier.

There is a kind of cot inside the back of the ambulance for me to lay down on. A thin, lightweight blanket to keep warm. I don't notice the many hands and arms all but carrying me from the wheelchair to the cot. I just go wherever the voices tell me to go, move wherever the hands put me.

Dr. Lorigan helps pass the bags into the ambulance.

"Safe travels," he says. "Godspeed."

I rub my eyes with my knuckles. It's impossible to make the cot as comfortable as the bed I'd just left, so I just give up and pull the blanket over me. It is strange at first, lying flat on my back in a moving vehicle. No sense of direction, no idea where we're going except for what I can see of the night sky outside the narrow back windows, turns and bumps that seem all backwards and spun around.

Streetlights pass by slowly, steadily picking up speed, then snapping past until my eyes stop trying to chase them. Deep, shallow breaths. A light, tentative sleep.

I'm sure it is the absence of movement, the absence of noise, that wakes me less than an hour later. The bright wash of lights, as if we're in a covered parking lot. A sleepy, fuzzy brain, trying to make sense of the situation. It doesn't seem like we've been on the road long enough to be in London already.

"*Whuzziza?*" I ask nobody in particular.

"Shh," Mom says. "Go back to sleep."

Propped up on my elbows, now, blinking through the harsh lights.

"Hurr," I manage to say, more exhale than anything else. "Hurrwethur?"

"No," she says. "We've stopped. There was a problem. Something with the transmission, I think. We've stopped. They've called it in, and we're waiting for another ambulance to take us the rest of the way. Shouldn't be much more than another hour." I'm so exhausted. I can barely keep my eyes open.

"Timeizzit," I ask.

"Late," Mom says. "Very late."

* * *

I have no idea what time it was when we'd eventually got started again, how much time was wasted dealing with mechanical problems in the middle of the night. I'm awake now, though. We're on the move and the stars appear to be long gone. Is it already almost dawn? Had we spent that much time getting nowhere in a broken-down ambulance?

There must have been a sleepy, zombie-like shuffle between vehicles. Two new medics – a driver and a navigator — and then our supplies and bags hastily moved from the back of one ambulance to the back of the other. As far as I'm aware, I'm the only one who's been getting any semblance of sleep the whole night.

It can't be getting light already. We should have been at Heathrow before now. Mom hates being late. She hates flying and she hates to be late, and we've lost our comfortable cushion for getting into London. There's still so much to do and hardly any time: first, I'll need to be examined by airline physicians. That's the easy part. She needs to get us checked in, going through customs, passports, talking with the airline about getting me on board the airplane before anybody else so I can get all settled in.

My vitals still need to be monitored every hour or so—and my current status is going to need to be conveyed to the airline, too. Looks like one of my bags of blood is empty. We'll have to replace that with a new bag, cold and dark, retrieved from a small blue cooler on the floor. Any time for breakfast? Doubtful.

This will be down to the wire.

After trying to sit up a bit and shake off my fatigue, another problem quickly becomes apparent: instead of avoiding the heavy morning traffic, we've run straight into it. I have no concept of how far away we are, but we're slowing to a stop and I don't see any airplanes. We do not have time for this.

I'm getting nervous now, too. Part of my brain pictures the 747 lifting off into the morning sky while we chase after it on the runway, but another part is convinced that the plane wouldn't just take off without us. I'm precious cargo, aren't I? We have a schedule to keep. I know that the airline does, too, but they can't just take off without us, can they? I mean: medical emergency and all that?

My limited understanding of my situation is that time, in the truest sense, is a luxury that we can't afford. I'd already waited long enough before going to the hospital in the first place, and even though it's only been just about ten days since I was scared enough about my symptoms to write them down, that's ten fucking days earlier that we could have started treatment.

Every day matters. Every hour counts. This is a race. If we miss this flight, I don't know how much longer that pushes everything back. Two days? Five?

I'm not sure who mentioned something to the driver, or if the growing sense of unease from the back of the ambulance was a palpable thing. It's likely nothing more than a collective awareness that *this simply would not do.*

"You're going to want to hold onto something," said the medic who was sitting where it had taken me months not to expect a steering wheel — one of the first times where I'd really felt "at home" during my stay in England was when I would be talking with friends, not paying any attention to what I was doing, and I'd correctly walk up to the passenger side of a vehicle. And then there are lights, and a siren, and we are moving again.

It's remarkable, the skill on display during our stretch run to Heathrow, the kind of thing that you find yourself enjoying more than you probably should, you know, given your condition. Bleeding a lot, remember? Car crashes are not friendly for people without platelets.

The two medics work in tandem: one aggressively driving and occasionally laying on the horn, the other constantly scanning the motorway, sometimes even leaning out his window, one hand firmly grasping an inside handle, waving and pointing and yelling.

Our driver *creates* lanes. He uses the shoulder when necessary. He slices his way through what seems, looking backward through the windows, to be nothing more than a four-lane parking lot. More horn, squeezing past slow-moving morning drivers, threading the needle all the way to Heathrow.

We actually make it! We're not here with anything approaching the buffer we'd been expecting when we left Lancaster, but at least we've made it. We have an hour or so left before takeoff. Time enough for one last swap of a now empty bag of blood for another new one, followed by hugs and kisses for Mom as we drop her off at the terminal with promises to meet on board as soon as we're done meeting with the United Airlines physicians, somewhere else in the airport.

We get to the infirmary with no difficulty. Once there, I notice a slight rash, warm, on the back of my hand. It's near where my stupidly painful IV needle has been providing blood to me all night.

"What is this?" I ask.

My RAF doctor looks at it. "Looks like a reaction," he says, reaching into one of his bags for a needle of sorts.

The rash spreads up my arm. My neck is flush now, too. My back. My doctor quickly wipes off a spot on my arm and plunges a drug into my veins. Stomach cramps kick in almost immediately. I don't know if that's from the drug he just gave me, or maybe a bad batch of blood? Does blood go bad? Is that even a thing? It's like knives in my abdomen!

Several people help me onto a table. White curtains are drawn around me. The RAF nurse is holding my hands and I'm trying to breathe and there are people shouting acronyms that don't make any sense to me.

"We're going to lift you now," somebody says, and then I'm on wheels and back into the back of the ambulance. Luggage is tossed inside. My doctor is next to me, my nurse is working with bags attached somewhere above me. The door closes.

"We can't fly you out now," the doctor says. "There's a hospital not far from here. We'll take you there until this reaction settles down."

* * *

It's freezing! It's not Minnesota cold here, but England can still get pretty frigid in these dwindling days of winter. I am absolutely not dressed for this, and I can't get warm.

My shirt's been removed so my doctor can run lines, take temperatures, do whatever it is that doctors do for patients in the back of ambulances tearing through London. There's no heat, at least none that I can feel. I'm curled up all fetal position, shivering, and I can't get warm. I feel like I need to stretch my legs out for some reason — to make it easier to administer whatever new drugs need to be administered, maybe?

I *still* haven't learned anything. There hasn't been time to research leukemia since I was diagnosed and I don't know if this is what it's supposed to be like. I'm so hot right now and I don't understand because I was freezing only a few seconds ago. And I'm trying to remember to breathe but my stomach hurts too much to think about anything else.

Is this what it's going to be like? Is this what I'm going to go through to get well? It scares me that it might be, and it scares me more that I have absolutely no idea what to expect.

I'm all turned around. The plan was Lancaster to Heathrow to Seattle. Hospital to Airport to Airport to Hospital. Very simple. But now I'm somewhere in London, driving someplace that wasn't part of the plan, missing an airplane that was. I can't figure out where we're going. I can't even form a cohesive sentence to ask the people around me about the new plan of action.

And Mom! Who's going to tell Mom that I'm not on the plane? How will she find me? What if she's already flying back to Seattle without me? Would they have done that? Would they have just taken off and left me here in London?

CHAPTER 10

They've given me a thin blanket, at least, standard hospital issue, after they'd wheeled me into the busy emergency room. Brick walls, linoleum floors. Activity all around. Surprisingly, thankfully, the stabbing pain in my stomach has already started to subside. It's manageable. Whatever meds my doctor had given me back at the airport must have kicked in. Most of the discomfort, now, comes from the fact that I haven't moved too far from the doors, and cold air continues to blast into the room.

I'm not *exactly* in the emergency room. See, there are all sorts of sick people in emergency rooms. Coughing, sneezing, wiping their hands on door handles or couch cushions or whatever. When your immune system isn't doing much of anything in the way of fighting infections on its own, it is not a good idea to place yourself into the middle of that environment.

In many ways, I'm already starting to learn, a hospital is the absolute worst place to be when you've got leukemia. But a hospital is also the absolute best place to be, for obvious reasons. Leukemia can be pretty fucked up that way.

I'm up against a far wall in this kind of a wide passageway, probably closer to the curb outside than the front desk inside, with thick brick walls and sliding glass doors on either side of my gurney. And those doors just keep on *opening*. My doctor is inside sorting out details of my unexpected arrival. He'd had my mother paged at the airport, earlier, as soon as we'd arrived at the hospital. My nurse stands next to me, very close by, casting protective glances at the people coming and going all around us. She tells me that my mom would be coming soon. Not to worry.

"They can't move you yet," she tells me, again, after I ask her why we're still waiting here. "You're not exactly a run-of-the-mill patient, now are you? We've got to make sure they can set aside a room for you, a clean one, disinfected. Isolated. That's going to take a little time yet."

"Don't they have any *temporary* isolated rooms? Someplace warmer, maybe?"

"Do you want me to see if I can get another blanket for you? Are you cold?"

"No," I say. "I mean, yes. Please. If they have one. Can you find out how much longer it will be?"

She smiles.

"Yes, of course. I'm sure I can find something. I'll be back in a moment."

And so after all of this movement from last night, all of this rushing to make it to the airport on time, all of this worry, there's nothing left for me to do but wait.

The extra blanket helps, when my nurse finally returns, but not much. I'm getting sleepy again. The cold isn't quite as bad when sleep beckons. I roll onto my side, bring my knees up close to my chest, putting the sliding doors at my back. I really should turn around to face the cold air, so I don't have to keep lifting my head every time I hear the doors whoosh open, hoping to see Mom coming through them. It takes a lot of effort to keep looking up. Pretty soon I just close my eyes for a second or two, trusting that things will work out.

When I wake up, who knows how many hours later, I'm in a new bed in a narrow room. Mom is in a chair pulled up next to me. My left hand dangles over the edge, wrapped up within both of hers.

* * *

This brief hospital stay in London is as good a place as any for a rapidly-edited montage. No words necessary, saving the cost of paying actors and actresses portraying the hospital staff for speaking lines in what, ultimately, will be a cameo appearance in my life.

We start with a shot of the hands. Mom holding mine. Maybe the camera blurs, or maybe it's a slow fade to black. Something cinematic and appropriate. Time to kick the soundtrack in again at this point, another song inexorably linked to my months in Lancaster, and to my rapid departure: *This Corrosion*, by The Sisters of Mercy.

We may have to work on a special, shortened re-mix, because the whole point of the montage in the first place is that while there is activity in that London hospital — doctors doctoring, nurses nursing, mothers mothering — it is neither a beginning nor an end.

It's an unwanted and unexpected two day transition between where I was and where I needed to be. We've stopped moving, and that's a little troubling. For the first time in about a week, there is nothing to do except wait until Saturday, when the next flight — Pan Am this time — will carry us across the Atlantic.

No fade to black: a quick cut after the hands, to an aerial, top-down view. Stop-motion photography, here, almost, meant to compare and contrast my sudden inertia with the ongoing hustle and bustle both inside and outside my body. There is a camera on a boom where the ceiling would be in this tiny room. I will be motionless, for the most part, tossing and turning occasionally in the bed. I don't get up much. Time passes. People enter and exit. They blur around the edges. Strips of sunlight crawl up the far wall, then disappear, overpowered by fluorescents. Food is brought to me, consumed, discarded. You can catch the back beat, the steady bass, and it almost feels like a dance. The camera has been moving steadily closer to my chest. The lighting appears to change again, daylight, maybe, gray and muted. It never gets completely dark, and I am never without company. The camera is close enough, now, that everything happening around me is nameless, faceless, a blur of hands with thermometers and blood pressure cuffs and tiny paper cups filled with medicine, needles and vials, blankets and pillows. The slow, inexorable drip of clear liquid from a bag above my head, down a plastic tube, winding into my arm.

The camera follows the tube, loses focus, then shoots into my body. Inside my bloodstream. I don't know that we need to show good blood versus bad blood, or what that would even look like. What the budget would be for the necessary special effects. We know there's bad blood in there; perhaps that's enough. Immature blood cells. There's music, and a steady beat, like a heartbeat, or a pulse.

We should let the camera linger somewhat. It is calm here, inside my body. Blood is pumping. Things appear to be working, even though they're not. The chorus repeats itself in the background. Over and over, like a hymn.

We are still so optimistic. That's how these two days close out. It's not boundless, or silly, or crazy optimism. I'm trying to keep myself grounded as I reflect on the days ahead and I can't help but feel happy. I'm looking forward to getting home. I'm looking forward to getting on an airplane soon — the beginning of my journey, really, although in many ways it feels like the end.

CHAPTER 11

There are so many differences between my two ambulance rides to Heathrow that it is impossible to draw a fair comparison between them. Most importantly, absolutely nothing goes wrong — *finally* — on my short trip from the London hospital. No blood transfusions, no emergency stops, no rush hour sirens blaring, and best of all, no sudden stabbing stomach pains.

Because we're already so close to the airport, the airline doctors have verified my readiness before we'd even checked out of the hospital room. One less wrinkle to fret about. There were no handshakes as they'd walked into my room earlier in the day: just tight smiles, a few questions for me, a few more for my doctor, all professional and courteous (*friendly, even*) while ticking boxes and writing notes on a clipboard.

The ambulance does not take us to the little-known Heathrow infirmary this time. Instead, we drive right onto the tarmac, right up to the plane. Wish I'd had a better view from the sheltered back of the vehicle, to see if there were chain link fences or barbed wire, or if it was just like any other service road. Luggage trucks and food trucks and me, all getting ready to be loaded directly onto a freshly refueled jet.

And while my health may have been vetted by the airline, there is still the simple matter of airport security. This is something they take very seriously in England.

A uniformed guard had been scheduled to meet our ambulance. He's wearing some kind of army uniform; something much more significant than the more traditional "rent-a-cop" airport security I'm used to. He's wearing camouflage fatigues, thick black boots, an M-16 slung over his left shoulder. Definitely military.

The four of us filter out onto the damp pavement: Mom, the RAF doctor and nurse, and me. I'm in a wheelchair. The ambulance driver transfers everything from the ambulance to the ground next to us: suitcases, overnight bags, cardboard boxes, rugged tackle box looking things, and two small coolers.

Paperwork exchanges hands. Passports, tickets, medical references, signatures from Pan Am physicians. The guard slowly looks through these, occasionally glancing over at me. Serious. Sharp. Mom's passport is less than a week old. He examines everything carefully.

"What's in the coolers?" he asks. A formality, I think, a casual question about the piles of obvious medical supplies that had formed nearby.

"Plastique," my doctor smiles. My *Royal Air Force* doctor.

The guard doesn't exactly straighten his posture — he was pretty rigid already — but he's noticeably on edge now.

"Pardon me?"

"Umm..." my doctor begins. "I was just..."

This is the last thing we need. I mean, there are *lots* of things that could be worse than this, big scheme of things, but I can't think of anything right now that would be more awful than spending a few hours in some back room of the airport, surrounded by even more guards and guns, a desk lamp shining into my eyes while good cop and bad cop take turns getting information out of me.

"Open them," the guard says. The assault rifle has somehow moved into his hands. He uses the barrel to point to the blue and white coolers. My doctor continues to stammer as he fumbles through his gear.

"Obviously medical supplies, just joking, blood, see, in case he needs another transfusion, this one, too, I'm sorry, really terribly sorry, just a bad joke, nothing here but medical supplies, obviously."

"I shouldn't need to explain to you the gravity of what you just said."

Please let us get on this plane. Please don't let a stupid joke prevent us from boarding. I need to get home. Please don't send me back. Please.

"I know," my doctor says. Penitent. Remorseful. "I really didn't mean it. It was just ..."

"Just a bad idea."

"I know."

Please, please, please.

"Just go," the guard says, left thumb pointing back over his shoulder to our plane. "Go."

* * *

We enter the plane through a door about halfway down the fuselage, somewhat behind the wing, on the left-hand side. Do airplanes have port and starboard? If you were inside, and you stood facing toward the front of the plane, we came in from the left, well past the main passenger entrance near the nose.

It's a pretty standard 747 layout. Two seats against the windows, a wide row of six (or maybe eight) in the middle, then another two window seats on the opposite side. Immediately across us from us, as we boarded, is a station for the flight attendants. It stretches across the middle of the plane, providing access to either aisle. There are two flight attendants here, putting away foil-wrapped meals, flipping switches on a long row of coffee pots, assessing inventory for the flight ahead.

One peels away to greet us. Short brown hair, a bright smile, a name tag that reads "Heather." She introduces herself and says that she's been expecting us. She's happy that Pan Am will be able to take me to Seattle. Heather is kind of beautiful. Her accent is as beautifully British as they come.

She places one hand lightly on my shoulder, a natural, practiced thing as the other hand points down the aisle to our seats nearby. I'd initially envisioned that I'd just have six seats all to myself, meaning an entire middle row that I could stretch out on if I'd wanted. Push up the armrests, grab some pillows and a blanket, kick back and enjoy the flight. Of course that's not the case. This is not the first time — and not nearly the last, I'd expect — that what I'd *imagined* would happen and what *actually* happened weren't even in the same hemisphere.

Heather had pointed to where three rows of window seats used to be. They'd been physically removed from the plane. A kind of temporary bed is bolted down, where the seats used to be, and a long metal rod runs parallel to the aisle. A makeshift cloth curtain, blue, is bunched up at one end. I'm guessing that will also be someplace where we can hang my IV and blood and platelets and such. Heather also explains that the three seats immediately across the aisle from my bed are set aside for the doctor, my nurse, and Mom. She tells me that there's an extra seat next to Mom's that I'm free to use anytime. They'd kept that one open for me.

I'm suddenly so nervous. I don't know why. This isn't what I'd expected. It's great. Really, truly, they've really done a great job of setting this plane up to get me across the Atlantic as comfortably as one could hope. And I'm excited to think about getting back home. It's all just so *real* now.

Things have been set in motion for me to get better. All of this is for me. Pan Am took six fucking seats out of this trans-Atlantic flight and built a bed so that I could have a comfortable and safe return to Seattle. This is really happening.

* * *

Lost in thought, I'm not paying much attention to the first passengers walking past our seats. Or my "bed," if you want to call it that. People of all shapes and sizes with their winter jackets and carry-on luggage file past. I'm acutely aware, suddenly, of how many people are coughing or sniffling. There's a low murmur of conversation but my ears are tuned into the sounds of other people's sickness. I double-check to make sure that my surgical mask is still in place.

Heads invariably turn to stare at me. I'm the worst kind of looky-loo accident slowing down boarding on my half of the plane. I'm not sure why I'd expected it to be anything different. Maybe it's because at least so far, everyone I've dealt with has been so courteous and so professional. It's been their *job* to accept me at face value. Doctors and sisters from the hospitals, ambulance drivers and medics, lab technicians, security guards, even my beautiful British flight attendant Heather didn't bat an eye at my situation.

And it's not as if I'm gaunt or stricken or oozing puss from my eyeballs or anything. It's not that. I'm feeling well rested and strong and as healthy as I've been in long while.

Can't argue with all the medical apparatus surrounding me, though. Or the cot that's been constructed specifically for me. Or the mask that I'm checking again, because I really don't want any of these germs to play havoc on what I already know is a barely functioning immune system. You can't help but notice the two Royal Air Force uniforms sitting across the aisle from me.

What on earth is wrong with him? I imagine people thinking as they walk past. Their voices are hushed as they move to their seats at the back of the plane. *Is he contagious? Why do they allow that sort of thing on board? I'm glad our seats are far away from him.*

As we lift off, settling in above the clouds for a smooth ride home, the imagined questions give way to unexpected comments. These are all well-intentioned, I know, but they don't make me feel like any less of a freak on display for the amusement of the rest of the passengers. If it wasn't me they were speaking to directly, it was with Mom, and the sentiment was consistently the same. *Oh, you poor thing. You poor, poor dear.*

Fear I could take. Loathing, even. It's easy to get angry at imagined ignorance. But *pity*? That's the last thing I want right now. I'm not dead yet.

✳ ✳ ✳

Grow up in the Pacific Northwest and you're afforded a built-in sense of direction, at least when the sun is out. Tourists don't necessarily know that the craggy jagged collection of almost-always-snow-covered mountains in the distance — *that way* — are the Olympic Mountains. Or those other hills — they must be hills, right? So clearly dwarfed by Mt. Rainier, or even Mt. Baker further north? They might not know at first sight that these are the Cascade Mountains. Olympics to your left, Cascades to your right, and you're facing north. The mountains guide you.

Tourists, though, look around and see the beauty of the mountains, but they're just that, snow-capped scenery providing a gorgeous backdrop to the lakes and evergreens. Both ranges run north and south: the Olympics to the west of Seattle, and the Cascades on the opposite side, creating a massive natural fence between the western and eastern halves of the state.

You grow up around these things and you always have at least a halfway decent chance of knowing where you're going. They are built-in navigation systems. You know the differences. You know that you may not be able to remember while driving downtown whether it's Pike or Pine that runs one way downhill towards the waterfront, but you will always be able to easily figure which direction you're headed, based on your view of the mountains.

I never knew how much I'd missed them until my freshman year at Carleton. It's not that Minnesota is completely flat — *look, my Midwestern friends would tell me, just a little defensive, there are hills all over the place* — it's just that nature opted for thousands of lakes instead of thousands of feet of mountain ranges. And the rolling hills that make up the miles of farmland surrounding Northfield are a poor substitute for even the non-mountainous ups and downs in and around Seattle. Parking brakes aren't a necessity in Minnesota. You don't even need to learn, counter-intuitively, that the wheel points away from the curb when you park uphill, into the curb on the downhill.

I suppose it's the same way with a lot of things: when you grow up with mountains, you don't always notice when they're with you, but it's immediately apparent when they're gone. For me, at least, there's something not quite right with an empty horizon.

To this day, I'm always alert for that last hour or so before landing at Sea-Tac. You're low enough to see the tree lines, the dark deep water of alpine lakes slowly passing underneath. Look left and Rainier dominates the view. Adams and poor, broken St. Helens peek out, too, with Hood visible further down the line.

The mountains bring me home.

✳ ✳ ✳

We wait until the rest of the passengers have disembarked before starting the process of getting off the plane. U.S. Customs had been informed of our arrival. Two officials meet us on board. There are more discussions. Our paperwork is carefully reviewed.

What little luggage any of us had is stowed all around us. Both coolers are lighter, now, after I'd received antibiotics and several more blood transfusions during the flight. The RAF doctor is professional and businesslike. Heather and some of the other flight crew wish me luck. There are brief, heartfelt hugs, followed by more good wishes, and then they deplane ahead of us.

We'll be leaving through the front of the plane like everybody else. Somebody has brought a wheelchair for me, waiting in the jetway. I'm not sure if it's from the hospital to get me quickly to the ambulance, or from Pan Am to finalize the transport of their cargo. Either way, I want to walk. I'm more than capable of walking on my own. The antibiotics feel good. The new blood in my body feels great. I don't need a wheelchair. I *don't*. I've got two working legs. I'm as well rested as I've been in months. Do they think I'm sick or something? That I can't manage a few hundred yards on my own in a friendly and familiar airport?

It's probably a look from Mom that settles me down. The expression on her face when she says "please, Robert, *please*, just do what they say."

Where landing at SeaTac is a welcome homecoming for me, a missing piece rolling softly into place — comfort, safety, stability, even with the promise of a scary and unknowable future — it is clearly something much different for her. She looks more exhausted than she did before we'd left London.

This is important for her. After these last few days, after completing this round trip from Seattle to England and back to get her only son, it's clear that it's more important to her that I use the wheelchair that's been provided for me than it is to me to walk into the terminal. I'd like to give her a chance to rest in this wheelchair, the way she looks now. But I think I understand. Sometimes it's important for parents to take care of their children, even adult children, and not the other way around.

This isn't a happy, festive homecoming. I need to remember why I'm back.

I'm in the wheelchair and Mom is behind me and somebody else is carrying our luggage and the RAF doctor and nurse are on the jetway next to us, asking for suggestions of places to see while they're in Seattle. They'll ride up with us in the ambulances to meet with my new doctors, briefly, before spending a day or two in town. After we get to the hospital, I doubt that I'll ever see either of them again.

* * *

The drive out of the airport is pretty much a south to north thing. We don't take the underground train to the main terminal, where hundreds (*thousands*) of complete strangers might cough or sneeze, and my lack of healthy white blood cells couldn't do much to protect me from infection. The ambulance is waiting not far from where the plane had landed. Immediate goal: keep contact with the rest of the world to a minimum. We take a service road out, stopping briefly at a security checkpoint before hitting a main road that I can never remember what to call other than "the road to the airport."

There isn't much to this road before it turns into I-405. A cloverleaf interchange, plus some confusing HOV lane changes, three lanes splitting off into three directions, north or south onto

Interstate 5, or continuing west into Renton. That's the way home. Take 405 a few more miles until you get to one of the downtown Renton exits, take your pick, then follow one of the main roads (usually Benson, but sometimes Petrovitsky) up the hill.

But I'm not going home. That's not the direction for me. I will be receiving treatment — whatever that means — at the University of Washington Medical Center. Roughly the mid-point of Lake Washington, north and a little west of downtown Seattle. Not too far from Dad and Jane's house on Phinney Ridge. The University has been expecting me for at least a few days now. I'm late. They have everything ready. They have been waiting.

We take the exit north onto I-5. The highway heads uphill for a bit, then jogs down and to the right as it crosses the Duwamish River, settling in for a long valley ride north. Boeing Corporate offices, then Boeing Field pass by on the left, with vast wide hangars and any number of 707s, 727s, or 747s just outside.

I'm stretched out in the back of the ambulance. There are two small square windows, one on each of the two rear doors. My view is limited, even if I wasn't laying down. I know that we're running parallel to Boeing not because I can see the vast airfield, but because I know this road. Home for the first time in almost six months, my senses are on high alert. I could probably keep my eyes closed the rest of the way and I'd still be able to picture the entire route.

The mountain is out. That's what we say when there are no clouds, no rain, affording often spectacular views of Mt. Rainier. I shouldn't be able to see it from this direction. We're traveling just a little north-east on this section of I-5, but I can see it behind us to the south-west, clearly, looming high above everything else. I'm fascinated by this unexpected view.

It's just because you're all turned around, I tell myself. *If you weren't in the back of an ambulance, you'd never see it this way.*

It's quiet. Pavement spins underneath. We're moving closer to the hospital, one mile at a time, and Mt. Rainier is frozen against the brilliant blue sky.

I know, I finally respond to myself. *That's what's so cool about it.*

✳ ✳ ✳

The ambulance takes me directly to the University of Washington Medical Center. We maintain the speed limit the entire way, no sirens needed. Traffic is light. The building itself a nondescript beige and gray and brown collection of buildings just across the street from Husky Stadium. Early spring flowers are planted in the boxes lining the circular drive.

Front door? Emergency entrance?

Probably we take the front. Too many sick people in the emergency room, and not as direct a route to my room on the sixth floor. Besides: this isn't an emergency. I'm expected.

Fast feet over concrete. Automatic doors opening automatically. Somebody in front of me, clearing the way, somebody else pushing from behind. Mom had been with me in the ambulance. She is at my side, now, as we move swiftly through an open lobby. An echo. Feet reverberating across tile, now. A gift shop passing by on one side, an espresso stand on the other.

People stand aside. Polite. Nobody stares. *Nothing to see here. Move along.*

The freight elevator is wide and deep. The walls are covered on three sides with a kind of dirty, padded quilt. It smells like a hospital. The whole place does. Whatever it is that hospitals smell like, closed windows, maybe, and cleaning supplies, and medicine, and whatever else that I never noticed when I was in Lancaster or London, this hospital has it.

The doors close behind us, and then we are up to the sixth floor. There is a desk with many people, working, writing, and I don't know how but Dad and Jane and Laura and Paul are already here, too — here with all these fluorescent lights and worn beige or tan or brown carpets leading down a maze of intersecting hallways. There are smiles from strangers, polite, inquisitive, white coats and introductions and a *we've been expecting you*, a moment or two of hesitation followed a collective *we're not exactly sure who's in charge now*, and then we're moving again, moving together down the nearest hallway, just two doors away.

The room is spacious. It has a stretch of windows along the west side, a view of pine trees, of Husky Stadium, of the Cascade Mountains in the distance. There is a bed that extends from the middle of the south wall. There is a sink near the bed, and a private bathroom near the sink, and chairs and low benches and a small table on wheels and a wall-mounted TV.

The room is wide and spacious and crowded. So many people standing at the edges of the walls, or at the foot of the bed, so many others coming inside with their faces and their hair and their light blue uniforms, their smiles and quiet voices, asking questions, writing on clipboards, then out, then in again. The only place for me is the bed. It adjusts. There are motors, and a collection of arrows that point this way for up or down, this way for sitting up or lying flat. My bed adjusts.

It is a blurry foggy blur, so many people here, suddenly, so many people in my room. *Yes.* That's it. Whatever else this room used to be, it is mine now.

CHAPTER 12

S cott and Blake arrive first, of all my friends. They burst
into the room with wide smiles. Scott's wearing khaki
shorts and an untucked tank top. Looks like he's just come
from the gym, shoulders and arms already a little sunburned, even
though it's barely March. He must have been in San Diego recently.
Blake is easily as big as Scott, strong, but with the more polished
wardrobe. Polo shirts, nice shoes, leather belts, everything all
precise and in place.

Scott gives my mom a big hug. He's done this for years. Not
sure how much of it is genuine and how much of it is an act that
he's perfected with my parents. He always calls my mom "Mrs.
Brown," always exceptionally polite and deferential. There's
laughter and loud voices. Big smiles. I'm not sure how they knew
to be here. Probably Laura gave Scott and Blake a phone call,
before I'd even left England. I've known both of them for years
— Blake since kindergarten, I think, although I skipped around to
a couple of different grade schools before we met up again at
Nelson Junior High. That's when I'd met Scott for the first time,
too. The three of us ran in different, but often overlapping crowds,
for much of seventh through tenth grades. We shared a number of

good friends: Jeff, Jackie, Shelby, Katie, Linda, Jimmy, Ron, Margarita, Carolyn. Circles of friends that I honestly felt on the outside looking in for much of high school as I worked on getting past some general shyness. That whole having lots of friends but not really feeling like you have any real best friends thing. Maybe that's just how we all feel at times?

What was it, junior year? Might have been senior year before things really started to click. Blake and I were in drama together. Scott and I worked after school at the Godfather's Pizza call center in downtown Renton, where we both looked forward to quiet nights without many orders so we could play cards, or Risk, or any number of games that fed both of our competitive natures. Neither of us liked to lose at anything, especially not to each other.

One day at school, our social studies teacher, Mr. Oyler, had asked Scott and I if we could help him with an experiment for one of his advanced classes. Later in the week, he was planning to give them a quiz. Didn't matter what the quiz was about. He wanted their attention to be focused on this surprise, fifteen-minute quiz.

What he wanted Scott and I to do, then, with permission from our teachers during that period, of course, was to start making some noise in the hallway. His students would be about five minutes into the quiz. He wanted us to argue. Loudly. And then come scuffling into his room, fighting, brawling, whatever. Mr. Oyler would rush over to break it up, horse-collaring us back out to the hallway and (presumably) to the principal's office. That's when his real quiz would begin: a test of situational awareness, of the accuracy of short-term memory when your attention is suddenly drawn to something new. He'd ask about what we were wearing, who came in first, what the fight was about, who hit who, and so on. Ten or fifteen conversational questions that he'd ask them after he returned to the classroom designed to seem impromptu, while still challenging their assumptions about how accurate their collective memories really were.

Scott and I wanted to get it right. We didn't want to half-ass this unusual assignment. So we consulted with our humanities and drama teacher, Bob. *How do we stage a believable fight?* We wanted our friends and classmates to think that it was real. We initially thought that we could throw a couple of punches, boxing, almost, like a couple of young prize fighters. Bob laughed. No way, he told us. No way does anybody telegraph punches like that in a real fight.

Bob helped us refine our script. We'd lay the groundwork earlier in the morning, getting surly with one another in the parking lot before school, complaining loudly to mutual friends about my totally bullshit interest in Scott's girlfriend. Then when it came time to act everything out later, the profanities came easily, shouted down the length of hallway in front of Mr. Oyler's class. The fight ended up being nothing more complicated than the two of us quickly closing the gap, grabbing, shoving, wrestling each other to the ground. Scott has easily fifty pounds of muscle mass on me. He started to pin me to the ground, gearing up to try throwing punch or two, but by that time Mr. Oyler had rushed over to break up our "fight."

It was the best. We became even better friends after that. I'm so glad that Scott and Blake are here right now. I've missed them. Their enthusiasm is contagious.

CHAPTER 13

Day blends into night. The lights dim in my room, but they don't go out all the way. There is still too much activity. Too many vital signs that need to be monitored every hour or two.

If I'm not already awake, then there is a gentle hand on my shoulder. I struggle to sit up. Propped on one elbow, perhaps. Two fingers lightly pressing at my wrist for six seconds. Then there is a thermometer. Then a snug wrap around the upper half of my arm. It gradually tightens, and then a cool stethoscope at the base of my elbow. Blood beats against the pressure. The wrap loosens, is stowed in a metal and plastic fixture attached to the wall behind me.

"Shh," my nurse says. "It's okay to lean back now, if you want."

The blood draw comes next. Four or five small glass vials are lined up neatly on a metal tray. They rest on top of a clean white towel. Each vial has a different colored cap.

"Lots of blood?" I ask.

"Lots of tests," my nurse says. She finds a vein. It's easy. I've got good veins. She doesn't need to look to long before finding a good spot on my left arm. The vials are vacuum sealed. This means that instead of four or five separate needles, like in Lancaster and London, it will only take a single poke to fill all the vials. There's a kind of open-ended attachment at the opposite end of the needle. The sharp end goes in. As soon as one of the vials snaps into place, upside down, the seal on the cap is broken and a tiny jet of blood spurts against the glass inside.

"*Cool*," I say. "They didn't have this in England."

My nurse nods. Her name is Anne. I'm trying to pay better attention to these things, now. I need to remember the names of the people who are going to help me get well.

"Yes," Anne says, a little distracted. She holds the needle in my arm with one hand and swaps out vials with the other. When the last vial is returned to the tray, she takes the needle out, wipes my skin again, and then tapes over it with a clean gauze.

"We won't be doing this too much longer, though," she says.

"What do you mean? No more tests?"

"No, it's not that. We just don't want to stick you any more than we have to."

"Oh. Well, it's not too bad."

She smiles.

"It'll get better. Tomorrow you'll be getting a Hickman catheter. No more needles."

"A what?"

"A Hickman catheter," she says. "A way for us to do blood draws, but also to get medicine into your system. Think of it as a kind of a permanent needle. Your doctors will explain it all to you in the morning. Try to get some rest, now."

✳ ✳ ✳

"The chemotherapy will be very strong," Dr. Collins tells me the next morning.

Dad and Jane are here, too, drinking good cups of coffee in the seats by my window. There is soft light on an otherwise overcast morning. It is Sunday, March 4th. This time yesterday, I was still in England. A little over a week ago and I was standing stupidly over a toilet bowl, watching it turn red.

Dr. Collins has been telling us about the catheter that will be inserted into my chest later in the day. "The chemotherapy will be strong," she says. "We'll assume it's chemotherapy for now, pending the results of another bone marrow aspirate tomorrow. Regardless, you'll be needing a Hickman catheter."

I'm barely half awake. Basic physics again. A body in motion continues in motion, except that I've stopped moving now, exactly where I need to be. And as much as I might want to put a brave face on it, leukemia really does wipe you out. Jet lagging, the emotional high of being home again, next to no healthy white blood cells remaining, a restless night in a strange bed with nurses waking me up every few hours, all of it means I'm spent. I know that this information is important, that I should be awake enough to be able to ask questions about all the things that will be happening to my body. I will need to be my own best advocate. But it's a struggle just to keep my eyes open while Dr. Collins is talking to me.

"Slow down, please," Jane asks. She is taking notes on a small yellow notepad. "The catheter? This is absolutely necessary? Robert needs this first?"

"Yes. The chemotherapy will be strong. It would tear his veins apart if we ran it through his arm. To say nothing of the other supporting antibiotics and blood draws that he'll be receiving. The catheter acts as a main line for us. It's an indispensable part of his treatment.

"You're very lucky, actually," Dr. Collins says to me. "Dr. Hickman works at the hospital here. He'll be putting yours in. It's a point of professional pride for him to put them in for our cancer patients. You'll be in best possible hands."

I nod. Dad or maybe Jane ask more follow-up questions. They will be my voice today. Jane wants more details about the procedure itself. Dr. Collins stands next to my bed. She touches a spot on the right-hand side of my chest.

"The catheter itself is essentially a thin plastic tube. You won't need anything more than a local anesthetic. Dr. Hickman will make one small incision here, and another, here." She traces a line almost up to my collar bone. "He'll guide one end of the catheter into your subclavian artery. It's a good, big vein for the chemo to enter your system, and for us to have access to everything we need. The other end of the catheter will come out of the middle of your chest, here. That's where your nurses will draw blood from now on."

My parents ask if there are any concerns about how much I've been bleeding but I just mumble something to Dr. Collins along the lines of "sounds good."

Everything sounds good at this point. I don't know anything about anything, and I have placed immediate, absolute trust in the people caring for me. My doctors could recommend running naked through the hallways, waving pom-poms, shouting *out, leukemia, out, geee-tttt OUT!* and I would cheerfully agree, only asking if I needed to find the pom-poms on my own — and what color? — or would the hospital be providing them for me?

* * *

Dr. Hickman is a kind-looking man, whitish hair, glasses, older than my dad, definitely, but hard to tell by how much. He smiles when we arrive. Dad had brought me down in a wheelchair, guided by one of the nurses from my floor. Dr. Hickman smiles and reaches out to shake Dad's hand. He pauses when I extend mine.

Even though he'll be putting in my catheter (*his* catheter?), he hasn't scrubbed yet, and he's cognizant of my condition. The rules are clear: nobody touches my skin unless they've washed their hands first. No exceptions.

"Pleased to meet you, Robert," he says, hands clasped behind his back. "That's my name, too. Great name." He nods toward my father. "It's good of your brother to come down, too."

We laugh together. It'll be cool. Nothing to worry about. Dr. Hickman is busy talking and cleaning, going through the specifics of the procedure for us. Nurses set equipment out onto tables set on wheels. Dad helps me onto a long table. My shirt comes off. Somebody points out the catheter itself. Looks simple enough: just a long, thin, white plastic tube that ends in a Y. Some kind of plastic clamps or something — one red, one white — on each end of the Y.

Gloves snap into place, and surgical masks, and a bright light shines overhead. We're quickly into this thing. Dad's still here, which is good, and although it seemed like a flurry of activity with nurses in and out of the room, maybe it was just the one nurse all along. My chest is wiped down with a cold swab. It is smeared orange. Several white towels are draped over my chest, horizontal, vertical, horizontal. I try to sit up, but Dr. Hickman is calm, soothing, saying "lay down, son."

Like other doctors before and after him, he says "little stick here" before injecting a dose of anesthetic. Maybe a couple of little sticks. Like bee stings. Then "tell me about England," or "crazy weather lately," or "so what kinds of things do you and your brother do for fun," or any number of distracting conversations until the anesthesia sets in and the prep work has been finished and there's no turning back.

It's a simple procedure. Dr. Hickman could probably do these in his sleep. And everybody is right when they say I won't feel a thing, don't even know when he's cut into my chest except that the blood spilling out tickles a bit.

And *fuck*!

Nobody mentioned the pressure. Or maybe they did but I just ignored the whole thing. Maybe I heard the simple part: two incisions, insert catheter here, done. Of course the catheter doesn't get from the middle of my chest up to my collarbone by itself. There's flesh there, and tissue. It feels like Dr. Hickman is kneeling down on my chest, both hands and a knee and a small truck, pushing a six-foot wide galvanized steel pipe up through my torso.

I'm gasping for air. Am I gasping for air? I must be. There's a large circus animal standing on my chest. Two. *Five*! How could it not be hard to breath?

"You're doing great, Robert, just ... a little ... more. There. All done." He smiles, unsnaps his gloves, removes his mask, smiles again, this time so I can see it. He explains that my chest will probably be sore for at least a couple of days, what with the pressure and all, and maybe some bruising, something to keep an eye on.

"Thanks," I say, blinking away tears. "Thanks. That wasn't so bad."

✳ ✳ ✳

When I return to my room, a new nurse takes an immediate interest in the Hickman. It sprouts all Y-shaped from the lower part of my chest. A square piece of gauze covers the entry point, taped on all four sides. Another smaller bandage sits just below my collarbone — the initial incision, I think, or maybe a cut where Dr. Hickman guided the tube into place.

Already my chest is swelling a bit. It's already a little bruised.

"Hmm," my nurse says, peeling away the tape. "Let's keep an eye on this, just to be safe." She takes a marker and writes on my chest, tracing the outline of the bruise. The gauze is already bloody, so she replaces it with a fresh square.

"We'll just keep an eye on this," she says.

I continue to bleed through the night. By four in the morning, the bruise has spread across almost the entire right side of my body. Blood collects in a purplish pool underneath my right arm. The gauze needs to be changed repeatedly.

One of the overnight nurses brings in what looks like an ankle weight. It's essentially a soft nylon bag, filled with sand or something, I don't know, used so patients can get some arm or leg exercises without requiring bulky weights.

"Here," she says. "Put this on your chest. It might be a little uncomfortable, but we really need to put some pressure on that site."

"That's fine," I say, remembering a similar need in Lancaster, and the way we'd improvised that, too. When morning finally arrives, Dr. Collins takes a studious look at the site of my Hickman catheter.

"You're bleeding a lot on us here, Robert," she says.

"Yeah," I say. I want to tell her how cool it is, how the bottom of my right arm is all purple and over-sized, or how tough it's going to be to look good on the beach this summer with all the extra black and blue running along my side. I figure it's best if I don't crack any jokes this early. She'll know anyway: I'm not making jokes to be funny. I'm making jokes because I'm scared.

A half-dozen other doctors form a semicircle around my bed. Dr. Collins sits next to me to get a closer look at the bruising.

"This weight?" she asks, setting it aside. "You kept this on your chest overnight?"

"Yep. The whole night."

"Any discomfort?"

"A little, but not too bad," I say. Not exactly the truth, but good enough for now.

Checking underneath the dressing, she finds that it's bloody once again.

✳ ✳ ✳

Platelets help your blood to clot. They thicken it, I suppose, like corn syrup or something. If you're in a hospital, and they're looking for this sort of thing, you can find out exactly how many platelets a person has coursing around their bloodstream. One of many components of healthy blood that are, apparently, easy enough to count with the right tests.

Mine are low. Silly low. Slap on the forehead "duh" kind of low when you look at how quickly and profusely I would bleed when given the chance. We'll pick a number to pin on the wall. Let's say 400,000. That's the number — the "count" — you might expect to find in your average Joe Healthy Guy. It's okay to be a little lower. Three hundred thousand is fine. Two hundred thousand is, too, even down to, say 150,000 or so. Anything lower than that should be cause for concern. But there's a wide range that can be considered healthy: 150k to 400k. They're only numbers. But numbers matter.

My count? My magic number that only matters when compared with the baseline? *30,000.* So far below the line that it's dangerously funny. No. This is serious.

It's no wonder my chest is all black and blue and swollen. And not just my chest anymore: the bruising has spread from my chest to my lower back. When I take off my shirt, the entire right half of my body, from Hickman to my waist, has been engulfed by a massive bruise.

Hence the almost immediate arrival of a steady stream of small blackish-purple bags that would take their place with many others on the top of my rolling metal cart. Bags filled with platelets keep arriving and I keep bleeding. I would bleed more without them, I'm sure, but even still, the donations are only so effective. They never help raise my counts in any significant way, and they only help a little with the bleeding and bruising. I need *my* platelets back. My blood counts need to be mine again.

* * *

"What's that?" I ask. It's early morning. One of my nurses — Cindy, this time, who I remember being here when I'd first arrived on Saturday — is inserting a needle into one of my free Hickman ports. There is a clear liquid. She pushes it in slowly.

"Heparin," she says. "It's a blood thinner. It'll help make sure that your blood doesn't clot."

"I thought my blood was already too thin. Isn't that what the platelets are supposed to be doing? Making my blood thicker again?"

"Yes, but there's a balance. We need to get control of all this bleeding, which is where the platelets come in, but blood clots are bad, too."

"So because of this," I say, tapping the freshly-replaced gauze on my chest, "I'm obviously bleeding too much. These platelets should help with that. I get that. But they might give me blood clots, too? So we put in something to make sure that doesn't happen?"

"Yes," she says. The plunger is empty.

"But I'll still need more platelets to help stop the bleeding, right? At least until I get mine back. And more Heparin, too? Then maybe more platelets again?"

"Exactly," Cindy says with a warm smile. "It's a balance."

CHAPTER 14

There's not enough time for all the tests that my team of physicians would like to run. The plan was to do another bone marrow biopsy today. I mean, we all know that I have leukemia. The results of various tests in England were abundantly clear. That's not the point of this additional biopsy.

Dr. Collins had explained that there's something about protocol, a specific and tested approach to my treatment, which requires a different battery of tests than what had been done in Lancaster. Honing in on the details. Leaving nothing to chance. It's not as if the University is being overly cautious, taking their sweet time. No. They want to be absolutely certain before moving forward. The plan was to do more tests today, including another sample of my bone marrow. My bleeding has changed all of that.

The Hickman, obviously, is critical to my ongoing care here. No way to get chemo into my body without it. To say nothing of the constant blood draws — and infusions — I'll likely need over the coming weeks. When it comes to my treatment, we're trying our best to keep from looking too far ahead — if there's a bone marrow transplant in my future, though, I think it would also to need to get into my body via this handy dandy Hickman catheter.

The things I'm learning: a bone marrow transplant isn't anything like what I'd imagined. The doctors don't actually take out my skeleton and replace it with a new one. Shocking, I know. No adamantium armor for me.

Marrow is soft. It's the stuff inside your bones, not the bones themselves. So, I've come to learn, a bone marrow transplant, as complicated and dangerous as it is, really means that there's just one more bag of stuff dripping into your body. The donated marrow drips down through the Hickman, and once it gets into your body, it knows how to get where it needs to be.

My Hickman catheter, then, helps us to plan ahead. I will need it for everything, even for things we're not sure I'm going to need, so there's no use apologizing for the state it's left me in. I can't even roll over in my sleep because I need to keep that ten-pound weight on my chest. My bruises continue to grow hourly. What to do, then?

Another hollow needle pushing through bone at the small of my back? After what we went through in England? After all the black and blue and purple emanating from where Dr. Hickman inserted his invention into my chest? No. Not this time. No more punctures, no more opportunities for bleeding.

Dr. Collins uses one of the chairs by the window. She pulls it into the middle of the room. It's mid-morning, now, on Monday the fifth day of March. Another gloomy, overcast day outside. Mom's taken the week off from work so she can spend most of the day at my bedside, holding my hand, opening cards and letters, reminding everybody that they need to wash their hands, first thing, before they come anywhere near me. It looks like her body has finally forgiven her for the recent time zone whiplash. Laura and Paul are both at their respective jobs. We'll update them later. Dad and Jane have brought coffee for everyone. One of my nurses had mentioned that I'll probably lose my appetite at some point, so a latte is welcome right now.

"We're going to do this by the book," Dr. Collins says. "Even without all the precision we'd like, there's still more than enough to move forward. Robert will follow a standard regimen of chemotherapy. We call this 'induction therapy.' Our primary goal, now, is to get you into remission."

"Remission? Is that the same as cured?" I ask.

"Not yet. I'll get to that soon. Remission is the first step, though. You don't get to cured without being in remission first."

Dr. Collins explains that after the team gets me to the much-desired remission, then we'll have had the opportunity to run more tests, to do the requisite detail-honing. She assures us that there will most certainly be follow up treatment. Until we know more, however, it's impossible to say whether that follow-up will be additional rounds of chemotherapy called "consolidation" (probably), or a bone marrow transplant (depends on a number of factors, not the least of which is whether or not my sister is a perfect match).

That's one of the main reasons for the Hickman. A large bag of rough-and-tumble chemicals will be placed at the top of a rolling cart. No, no. A cart isn't the right word. This thing has a display, and a battery, and it regulates the various speeds at which different antibiotics, blood, or chemicals will need to drip inside of me. Much better than gravity. Much more than just "a cart." Picture a metal coat rack on wheels, with an electronic display halfway up.

Standard protocol, to get this started, is one week of chemotherapy. Dr. Collins calls it "seven-and-three." A large-ish, heavy-ish, clear-ish bag will be placed on one of the free hooks at the top of my cart. A line runs down from the bag, through the electronic panel, and into one of the Hickman ports. Drops of chemo fall from the bag, one at a time, until it is empty. Slowly. Takes a day, maybe, to empty the bag. Once empty, it will be replaced by another bag.

"This chemical," Dr. Collins explains, "is called ara-C. It's standard. Very normal, very standard."

This is my chemical therapy. My chemo. This is how I will begin to get better: the bags of ara-C will drip and be replaced, drip, replace, for seven full days. At day five, though, a new bright red bag, much smaller than the ara-C, will be added to the top of the cart. There are plenty of hooks. There's lots of room. It, too, will feed into my Hickman catheter, directly into my subclavian artery, disseminate through my body however chemicals do that sort of thing.

Dr. Collins holds out both bags so we can see what they look like. The smaller one, she tells me, is called daunorubicin. This is the strong stuff. So potent, this particular part of my chemo, that it's only added to the mix for a few days at the end. It drips more slowly. You can watch the drops forming before they shoot down the clear plastic tube. I will be getting this for twenty-four hours a day as well, during the last three days of the week.

That's seven days of ara-C combined with three days of daunorubicin. *Seven-and -three*. This is our strategy. This is the plan. It's how we'll say "goodbye" to the defective, unhealthy, immature blast-producing bone marrow, and "hello" — *hopefully* — to strong, healthy, back-to-normal marrow.

"This is your protocol," Dr. Collins says. "After these seven days, we'll take a break. We'll let you recover. This is all standard, Robert. The chemo will continue to work well after we've stopped in a week. You'll continue to feel it. Most of your side effects will start kicking in then. We'll give it another week to keep working through your system. That means two weeks from today we'll do another bone marrow biopsy to confirm that you've made it into remission."

✳ ✳ ✳

These first days of chemo are a number of different things at the same time. On the one hand, there's little to no pain. The chemicals don't burn. I guess I'm surprised by that, given how much my nurses — Cindy and Anne, mostly, splitting the morning and evening shifts — had warned me about their potency. I can't feel them shredding my veins or anything. They're just these diligent workers, tiny, unseen, coursing through my body, on these myriad important search-and-destroy missions.

I also haven't been required to do anything. I'm being waited on hand and foot, it seems, meals brought on plastic trays, placed quietly on the far table if I'm sleeping, rolled right up over the adjustable bed if I'm awake.

There's a TV set on the far wall, and a remote control. But even that gets boring. When I'm not visiting with visitors, or watching television, or noticing raindrops forming on my window, it's really very quiet. This is one of the other things. Since I'm not actually doing anything — getting all these tests done for me, doctors and nurses so smiling and helpful, hands on my back helping me onto the scale, or the gurney, or the wheelchair, helping me to the bathroom, to the shower, just a walk down the hall, all these helping hands helping everywhere — much of my alone and awake time is an exercise in extreme boredom.

I do *not* want to let my imagination wander. I can imagine all sorts of terrible things. When it's three thirty in the morning and I'm wide awake because my body clock is all kinds of backward — light in the darkness, darkness when I'm expecting light, still not completely adjusted to Pacific instead of Greenwich Mean — and there's nothing on TV, and the visitors are long gone, I'm more than capable of imagining the worst of the worst. So I just don't.

Instead, I start thinking about getting back to Carleton in the fall. I have some work to do, still, to complete my credits for my final term at Lancaster. That's important. I'll think about getting through tomorrow, no matter what it brings.

And something else occurs to me during this week: how incredibly, unbelievably lucky I've been. I'm getting my chemo in probably one of the handful of best hospitals for this sort of thing in the entire country, if not the entire world, and it just happens to be where I grew up.

Word spreads. People know. Close family friends are some of the first to visit. They smile and wash their hands at my sink before approaching carefully with hugs and handshakes. Everyone is well past commenting on how much bigger, older, or more mature I look since the last time they saw me. It's also probably not appropriate, given where they're visiting me. I'm not always happy, don't necessarily have enough energy to keep conversations going. It's easy enough to just cut the visits short so that I can attend to a very important nap.

Scott, Blake, and other friends from high school are back frequently, too. It was great that they'd showed up on that first day, and I'm happy to see them again. Sometimes together, often alone. We do a great job of pretending like there's nothing to worry about, falling back into the kind of friendly banter we've always had together. They're here, though, almost daily. They show up.

They've obviously been sharing the news with other high school friends and teachers from Lindbergh. It's been a few years since graduation for most of us. Going to college in Minnesota means I've kind of fallen out of touch with more than a few friends here. But they, too, will be worried, and will call or just stop by. They bring cards and flowers — although, we all learn together, the flowers can't stay in my room. Suppressed immune system and all. Those go back out to the front desk, or they'll be shared with other patients on the floor who don't have the same issues I do.

There's laughter and smiles as we remember good times from high school together. It's tough to condense the past few years of college into "catch up conversations," and besides, there are obviously more important things to talk about.

Everybody is so thoughtful, and so concerned. I tell them as much of the truth as I know for any given moment: I'm doing well, and the chemo isn't too bad, but it is far too early to tell whether it's working or not. I'm just so happy to see them. I am so thankful for this instant support network. So lucky to have so many visitors multiple times throughout each day.

My days are both empty and full. There is a duality about everything, it seems, at once bad and good, energizing and exhausting.

* * *

One of many first things I do each morning is stand on a scale. Michele is about my age. She's studying at the UW. Part of her internship (*or maybe it's just a student work program*) is to wheel a large scale up and down the halls. The scale has hand grips, waist high, almost like a treadmill. My doctors want to make sure that I'm not losing too much weight, and Michele is here to check my numbers. Weight is something that needs to be monitored for all the patients on the sixth floor. Yet another number that must be written down, tracked and charted, searching for trends over time.

Sometimes I'm awake when she knocks on my door, sometimes not. She is very kind. She brings the scale close to my bed so I don't have to move too far, especially if I'm only just waking up. The hand rests are padded, which is nice. I don't have to lift my feet or anything. Just reach over from the bed, swing my bare feet to the scale, stand still for a few seconds, and then watch the numbers climb up from zero before slowing to a stop on a different number almost every day.

165 pounds is as good a reference point as any, my baseline weight when I'd first arrived. Immediately after I'd received my Hickman, after all the bleeding that followed, my numbers shot up. I'd extend my arms, pointing to the blood pooling into dark bruises

underneath my right arm, and Michele would nod while she confirmed what those meant to my weight.

She wrote down 175 last week. That's my high-water mark. The bleeding eventually slowed. My bruises had stopped growing. Things settled down.

We'd held steady for a few days after that, but once the effects of the chemo had started to kick in — and even more so, now that my appetite is completely gone — my numbers began to drop. Just like everything else, it seems, my weight has been trending downward. It's been a pound or two every day for the past week, and now I'm right back to where we'd started: 165 pounds.

We'll keep an eye on this. Michele will help me to monitor this particular number, but that's all we'll be able to do. I can't eat. There's no way I'll be able to maintain anything close to my baseline weight until I'm able to start consuming actual food again.

✳ ✳ ✳

I'm still feeling pretty solid. Relative term, of course, but I figure things could be a lot worse. My counts aren't coming back anytime soon, which is to be expected, but antibiotics and platelets can work wonders.

The chemo had stopped a couple of days ago.

Most mornings I'll shuffle over to my bathroom. When I was still in Lancaster, Gail had asked me what I'd really wanted for my time in the hospital, once I'd made it back home. Based on what I ended up wearing almost exclusively while in England — borrowed pajamas from the Royal Lancaster Infirmary — and because I usually just sleep in shorts and a tee-shirt, I'd told her that some real pajamas would be a welcome treat. One of the first things she'd done for me (after she came back, too) was to bring me three or four pairs of these really comfortable cotton pajamas. Pants and a button-up top. Classic. White, with thin blue stripes. I'll shuffle out of bed most mornings with my incredibly comfort able pajamas and my bare feet on the cool floor and I'll get my first puke of the day done and over with.

I'm not eating much. Haven't been eating much for days, now. It's one of the gradual things that are hard to put your finger on when it's happening — the slow disappearance of any sort of appetite, replaced with a constant uneasy emptiness and this taste like sucking on keys.

It's no big deal, I figure, *just part of the process.*

Sometimes I'll exacerbate my first morning vomit by drinking cold apple juice afterward. We all know what it does to my stomach. Cindy and Anne and Dr. Collins and my parents all tell me to let it get warm, at least, or to just drink water if I'm thirsty. I don't care. I *like* this apple juice, and I like it *cold*. For some reason, I can sort of taste it past all the metal in my mouth.

I know what happens next, too. I'm not stupid. Every day it's the same. The apple juice is cold and I slam it down in one ravenous gulp. When I feel my second puke of the day approaching, I politely excuse myself and close the bathroom door. I kneel on the floor. My stomach heaves. I use a square of toilet paper to wipe involuntary tears from my eyes, then wash my hands before returning to bed.

It's a routine. The chemo drips. It drips constantly. My appetite vanishes. Sometimes I have to take pills a second time if I throw up too quickly.

These things are normal, expected. The nausea is, of course, textbook. I'm hungry but I'm not and when I'm not I'll just throw up again anyway. I barely notice that I've stopped eating altogether. Those rare times when I feel hungry, my throat rebels against me, a gag reflex with almost any solids I attempt to force down.

We have the requisite discussions with my nutritionist. A new bag, bright yellow, is introduced at the top of my little buddy. "Bacon and eggs" is the joke, but it's actually called TPN: *Total Parenteral Nutrition*. All the many nutrients that I'm unable to get down my throat will now slide in through my handy, multi-purpose Hickman. These nutrients won't make the nausea go away. Oh, no. The chemo is dead set on still kicking me while I'm on my way down. My stomach is one of the unfortunate casualties in our war against leukemia. Now that I'm not eating, though, this large yellow bag of nutrition will ensure that I don't drop too much weight before I finally get out of the hospital. While I'm unable to eat anything, at least my "bacon and eggs" will provide some sustenance. I will need my strength in the days ahead.

I'm not trying to be glib about these things. When I say "it's no big deal," of course I don't mean that it's perfectly normal to wake up and vomit, then make my way to the bathroom every few hours throughout the day to just kneel in front of the toilet again and again, dry heaving nothing into nothing. Yes, that part of it absolutely sucks. It's really fucking shitty if you want the truth of it. I kind of hate how I feel.

But put it in context: I have leukemia. I've been receiving a controlled dose of poison nonstop for days in order to fight back. I'm not resting comfortably at home, nor am I anywhere close to the picture of health. It's not as if my puking throughout the day is somehow unexpected or out of the ordinary. I'm trying to stay big picture here.

These are known side effects. The chemo is harsh, and it makes me want to vomit. It creates this awful and persistent metallic taste in my mouth. So what? The chemo will also cure my leukemia. Sounds like a fair trade to me. The very definition of "short term pain, long term gain."

It doesn't take long before the falling out of hair really begins in earnest. I'll wake up and lift my head from my pillow to find clumps of left-behind hair. Or I'm napping in the middle of the day, only to roll over and taste hair in my mouth. In the shower, rubbing shampoo into my scalp, I'll wash my hands again to get all the hair out from between my fingers. It's falling fast.

A day or two of this and I've had enough. More than enough. Cindy has a set of clippers. Or she has access to some that are shared by the entire sixth floor. We set it to low. The lowest setting. What is that? One? Zero? As close to the scalp as you can get, as close to bald without actually shaving. Gone. Done. Good riddance. One more thing to trade away on my path to wellness.

* * *

My room is on the sixth floor of the University of Washington Medical Center, in the southeast wing. It's the cancer ward. The nurses are fantastic and well-trained. They pay attention to details. They provide an extraordinary amount of extraordinary care. When you approach the front desk, you will turn down the first hall immediately to your left. I am in the second room past the desk. I am close to everything.

The rules are strict, but a little different than what they were in England. Between Lancaster and London, the number one rule when I was outside my room was that I needed to wear a surgical mask. All sorts of badness could be transmitted through the air, especially within the confines of the hospital. Wearing the mask keeps the badness at bay. That was the theory.

Here, we are not so concerned with what I might happen to breathe while walking through the hallways — the off chance that somebody might sneeze and it might linger and then I might, maybe, get sick from that airborne whatever — as we are with physical touch. As long as hands are washed regularly (and always before touching me) the mask is all but irrelevant as long as I stay on this floor. Dr. Collins has given me permission to walk outside, if I want, but that's when the surgical mask would need to come back.

This freedom to move about — at least on my floor — is one of the reasons I try to get out and walk at least once a day, even if it's only a single lap. So what if I'm a little vain and don't want to be seen wearing a mask? I'm bald, barefoot, almost always in pajamas. I'm holding onto a rolling cart with one hand. My cart and I are always together, connected by plastic tubes. We go everywhere together. I've already taken to calling it my "Little Buddy," always holding up bags of blood and chemo and platelets, rolling with me, hanging out, making sure everything drips down just like it's supposed to. We are inseparable. It's got my chemo and a big bag of nutrients and other antibiotics and platelets hanging from the top, all dripping into the clear plastic tube stuck into my chest. There are visible bruises along my side, gathering at my waist. I am more than fine ambling up and down the halls like this. But ask me to wear a surgical mask? In *public*? The horror.

If I don't need to worry about anything other than washing my hands when I get back and making sure that nobody touches me — don't anybody come near me — then I'll walk around whenever I can.

Dr. Collins will scold me, of course, when I go barefoot. Broken glass will cut unprotected feet, and hospital floors might not always be spotless, and a certain cancer patient hasn't proven to a certain oncologist that his feet won't bleed all over the floor if flesh meets glass. I leave my slippers behind, for now. I'm a rebel. I'm dangerous. I know these floors are kept clean. I'm living a rebellious, slipper-less life on the dangerous edge, walking barefoot laps around 6 SE.

CHAPTER 15

Cindy is taking my pulse. Two fingers rest lightly on my left wrist. That's the side closest to the door. She watches the seconds tick past on one of the many cool watches she wears, big watch faces, bold colors. Her hand touches my wrist for six or twelve seconds.

"How's it?" I ask.

"Okay," Cindy says. She puts the back of her hand against my forehead. "Feeling warm again?"

"Not really. I mean, maybe a little."

The thermometer comes out. It's like a big battery in a blue plastic case. There's a thin metal rod attached to the case with a tightly wound cord. Cindy has been doing this a lot recently. We take my temperature much more frequently now, trying to gauge how often, and when (*so maybe we can begin to understand why*) my fevers come. She pushes the metal rod into an attachment on the side of the box; it comes back out with a clear plastic covering. More sanitary that way. It also means I won't taste the metal, not that it matters. *Everything* tastes like metal.

I'm not sure how long we keep it under my tongue. She holds the digital read-out so we can both watch it. It's easy to guess how high it will go based on how high it starts, and how fast the numbers change. I'm spending most of my time with temps well above 102. They rarely get lower, but often spike higher.

Cindy takes the thermometer out of my mouth and writes down a few numbers before moving past the foot of my bed on her way out the door. She touches the lower part of my leg, still buried underneath sheets and blankets. "Rest," she says.

Her presence is comforting, reassuring, steady. I don't know exactly where or when or how both Cindy and Anne became so important to me. Only through steady repetition was I able to even recognize my primary nurses. Only with time have I begun to understand how much I've come to rely on them.

Cindy arrives in the morning to check my vitals. She introduces herself every time until I remember. She always smiles. Black hair, slight build, fit. She is quick, and professional, and courteous, and beautiful. Young. Late twenties, maybe? She wears big watches in primary colors. Cindy moves with purpose throughout my room. She returns throughout the day, a bundle of energy, checking more vitals, hooking me up to another bag of platelets. She is there almost every morning. She works through the morning and into the afternoon, checking on me frequently.

Anne arrives in the evenings. There'd be a shift change sometime in the afternoon, the baton would be passed, and now Anne is the one checking vitals and replacing bags and helping with my meds. She has red hair, a smallish, slim build, and clearly athletic with her strong arms and wrists and hands. A little older than Cindy but not by much. Anne is quick to tease me, to rib me, to allow our conversations to descend into friendly banter.

This is my routine. Cindy takes care of me during the day, Anne at night. And even though there is often a third or fourth nurse working the overnight shift, my interaction with them is minimal. I'm sleeping somewhat regular hours, finally, and I trust that when I wake each morning, Cindy will be there to make things better.

CHAPTER 16

A thick manila envelope arrives with the mail. It's all multi-colored ink and smiley faces and hearts and shiny metallic stickers. Postmark is from Northfield, Minnesota, and the handwriting is so familiar.

Sophomore Year at Carleton: Ken, Tor, Adam and I are living together on the corner of third Musser. It's a lousy dorm, one of the worst on campus, tiny rooms, barren walls, but we're living together by *choice* instead of some random freshman room draw. We're the All I-90 room, starting with me on the far west in Seattle, picking up Adam in Pullman, Tor in Missoula, then continuing south and west until we get to Ken in Rapid City.

An interesting fact about Musser — other than the fact that it's this form-meets-function bland box of a dorm built in the sixties with a twin, Meyers, halfway across campus — is that in order to cram more rooms into the box, there are five single rooms per floor, two on each end, and an extra for the RA. One of the few dorms on campus where you could find a single. Linda lived in one of those: a no-bigger-than-a-walk-in-closet room to herself immediately across the hall from our quad.

I can so easily get sidetracked here, so easily remember how good it was for the four of us to have Linda so close, how good it was for her, too, going through some difficult times — her mother's battle with breast cancer — that we wouldn't know about until later in the fall. Aaron lived down the hall from us, too, a fortunate coincidence that has turned into a great friendship. A lot of good came from living in Musser last year.

I *loved* living there, okay, loved living with Tor and Ken and Adam, with Linda just across the hall. It was like we were five roommates, really, with the amount of time we'd either spend with her in her single, or she'd spend over in our room. Rooms, actually: the "quad" was nothing more than adjacent doubles with a connecting interior door. We'd bunked all four beds in the far room. In the other, our main room, our "entertaining" room, we'd made this sort of futon out of a turned-over bookcase and an extra mattress. We'd pushed this up against the window. It wasn't spacious, by any stretch, but it was home.

Spring term, Linda and I would crank the stereo. Fine Young Cannibals. *She Drives Me Crazy.* We'd jump up and down on the not at all bouncy futon, shouting at the top of our lungs. We'd open the window to let the fresh smell of spring into the room. We'd yell out the window. Amazing how good the departure of winter feels.

Our other spring term project last year took much, much longer than any of us expected. All the halls in Musser are lined with white tile. Like a bathroom. Not exactly the most aesthetically pleasing architecture, most certainly not the dorm featured in all the campus literature. The one saving grace was that there were half a dozen large bulletin boards, a good four feet tall, five feet long, three on each of side of the dorm. Between various door decorations and whatever people decided to put on the bulletin boards, it wasn't all *that* bad.

The big boards were a nice idea, but people crapped them up pretty quickly. I mean, even if somebody decided to cut out a whole bunch of photos from the latest J.Crew or Benetton catalog and pin them up, you wouldn't be surprised to see mustaches or other graffiti by the end of the weekend. It wasn't like the dorm was this horrible broken-down place. It's just that people didn't really care. You live there for a year, do your time, then move on to a better spot on campus.

I'm sure it was Linda's idea. We maybe came up with together one night, casually, all of us in our room, drinking whatever cheap case of beer we could pick up at the Muni. There was a board across the hall from our quad. We walked past it every day, every day thinking how much it sucked.

Inspiration strikes on a Friday night while picking at the edges of beer labels: we could do something cool. Something *different*. We could do something that nobody has ever done before, that would be amazing and artistic, and that drunk graffiti writers could respect. I'm absolutely certain that if it wasn't Linda's idea, then she was largely responsible for its implementation. We wrote a letter to the appropriate campus groups. We asked building maintenance to remove all the junky scraps of paper that tattered our board, and then please paint it white. We wanted a solid four-foot by five-foot rectangle of clean, unblemished promise. *A blank canvas.*

From there, we only ever ordered bottled beer for the weekends. We wanted variety. We wanted any number of different brands of beer: Pfeiffer, because it was dirt cheap, but also MGD, Kiran, Budweiser, Old Milwaukee, Coors, St. Pauli Girl. We started looking for cases of beer based not on the price per bottle, but on the colors and shape of the label.

On Saturdays and Sundays we'd walk our black plastic garbage cans down the hall to the shower. We filled them with halfway with lukewarm water, then brought them back down to our quad. Homework was done on the futon, or in the chairs lined up next to the bookshelves. We all shared the work. Empties were added to the garbage cans, left to soak for thirty minutes, maybe an hour. Labels were carefully peeled off, laid out along an empty bookshelf to dry. Some labels were more difficult than others. You had to be patient.

When the labels were dry, we'd glue them to the board. Patterns were formed. A Pfeiffer border. A large swirl of MGD labels. A checkerboard of Bud and Bud Light. We didn't have any kind of master plan as we began to glue the beer labels to the board, but we recognized how certain labels would dictate placement. It was a work in progress.

Nobody touched it. Nobody defaced it. This was a surprisingly brilliant, completely accidental strategy. Drunk college students living in a crappy dorm tend to break shit. But when they'd stumble up the stairs to third Musser and stumble even further down the hall to our collage, they were humbled. *It's beer, dude. It's beer ... and it's art ... and, fuck, dude, it's fucking beer.*

We'd drive down to the Muni with purpose near the end of the term. There were so many people involved, now. We'd all stand in front of the beer board — Ken, Adam, Tor, Aaron, his roommate Dave, Linda, Linda's best friend Karen — and we'd survey the patterns, keeping an eye on the decreasing amounts of white space. We'd think about how many cases we'd need, what brands to look for, as we invited more friends to another spring term party.

"Help us," we'd write. "Help us finish these cases of beer. Help us finish the mural."

On the bottom left side of the border, Brady carefully cut out the Pfeiffer wording from labels we'd pasted there. He filled the space with each of our names, hand-drawn to match the red script, something you probably wouldn't even notice unless you were looking for it. When it was finally finished, we felt we'd created a masterpiece.

I'm turning the manila envelope over in my hands, thinking about my friends in Minnesota. The envelope is thick and light. The handwriting definitely belongs to Linda. Winter term finals are wrapping up. If they haven't already, everybody's left campus for spring break. I don't expect anybody to call or write these days, either too busy studying, or too busy partying, so the thick envelope comes as a surprise.

I hope it's not cookies. I could imagine Linda had decided to stay up late one night, maybe calling Aaron or Tor or Karen to help bake chocolate chip cookies in the lounge. She'd done this often for us last year. My stomach is in no mood for such a sweet gesture.

It's a VHS tape. The spine reads *We Miss You, Robert!* Each letter is a different color. There's also a blank piece of paper with the same message spelled out in large letters (all blue this time), signed by Aaron, Linda, Tor, and Karen. Little hearts and cute smiley faces adorn everything.

I am so excited! *Thrilled.* Cards are great. Letters are fantastic. But nobody has ever made a video for me before. I don't have any idea what's on it. I can't wait to watch it. We pop it into the VCR.

There's no introduction, no fancy titles or soundtracks, just the tape popping and hissing to life, then a jarring hand-held view of friendly, familiar faces. Tor and Brady and Aaron are all in Linda and Karen's room. They're talking directly to the camera. They're talking to me, filling me in on important things (*like the surprising but not at all surprising fact that Tor and Linda have started dating earlier in the year*), and not-so-important things (*like the strange karate chop noises Brady made the night before last while walking back from a party at Hill House*).

It's maybe twenty, twenty-five minutes long. Karen and Linda share camera duties. They start in their room and give me a virtual tour of campus. They walk outside in the rain, stopping at the Libe, and Laird, moving to Nourse, then Evans. They stop people I know — and sometimes complete strangers — asking them to say something to the camera.

I'm crying and I'm laughing and I'm holding my breath, waiting to see who they might happen to bump into across campus. Linda and Karen do a goofy skit in Nourse Little Theatre where they both profess their undying love for me. Periodically they will break into a variation of Paula Abdul's *Opposites Attract*.

"We miss you, Robert. We really want you back!"

It is the best kind of medicine. It is instant healing.

CHAPTER 17

My room has become very homey. Cards and letters are pinned to one of two large corkboards opposite my bed, just below the TV. There's a *Far Side* calendar on the right-side corkboard. I've been using a fat permanent marker to cross out the days. I started by writing a big "X" across each day I've been here. Lately, I just scribble out the numbers. I make sure the black ink wipes out the dates entirely. It's as if these days are not only past, but that they never existed in the first place. You can't read the numbers unless you get up real close. You need to squint to decipher what's underneath the permanent ink.

There is a row of already opened bottles of pop on the small shelf that separates the two boards. Big bottles, two liters, all completely flat. My nutritionist had explained to the family that chemo would have an adverse effect on my appetite, and that drinking cold carbonated beverages might make the nausea worse. Mom had stopped by Safeway before one of her afternoon visits. She'd picked up several two-liter bottles of Dr. Pepper, Coke, Pepsi, and Mountain Dew. A sampler. We didn't know if I would even be able to taste the pop, so she'd hedged her bets. She'd lined the bottles on the shelf in my room and opened them all. She had wanted them to be ready for when I'd eventually lose my appetite.

What I could taste of them was horrible. Flat lukewarm pop, whether you've been getting chemo or not, just does not belong in anybody's system. The bottles stayed on the shelf, though, caps on, not getting any colder or more carbonated, in case I might suddenly start to like them in the weeks ahead.

There are no flowers. Not anymore. Hospital rules. It's too easy to catch an infection from real flowers. The room is kind of a mess. Not dorm room messy, with books and pens and loose change all over every available space on my desk, posters on the wall, dirty laundry piling up in my wardrobe, but a kind of lived-in, I've been in a hospital room for a couple of weeks kind of messy.

A few Mylar balloons drift lazily near the ceiling. The more comfortable chairs remain lined up against the window. Mom has brought one of the folding chairs next to my bed. Close. She's being doing this for a while now, staying close, holding my hand when I sleep. Sometimes we don't talk at all. Sometimes I'll do that thing I used to do when I was much younger, pretending to be asleep in the back seat of our old red Cutlass Supreme, my head nodding realistically with the motion of the road.

She cries a lot, sitting in that narrow folding chair, holding my hand. She will be sobbing and I won't know what to do or say. I will want to apologize, even though I know doing so will makes her sobs rack harder, feeling guilty that I'm feeling guilty. And so on. I'll do that thing, that thing I did when I was a kid. I'll end up drifting off anyway. I'm so exhausted. It's too easy. Pretending, sleeping, what's the difference?

Dr. Collins is here, too. She has been talking for a little while, explaining the results of my most recent bone marrow aspirate. I should pay attention to this. We're fourteen days into it, now, two full weeks after beginning my chemo.

It's mid-March. Today marks my third Monday at the University of Washington Medical Center. The great news is that my bleeding is no longer a concern. I'm still not producing any of my own platelets, but the almost daily infusion of other people's platelets — *you down with OPP?* — has been a tremendous help. The biopsy I'd had yesterday didn't require any of the extra care and concern like the one from Dr. Gorst in Lancaster.

While it's fantastic that I'm less likely to bleed out, that's not the end game. It's a step along the way. Some things *should* be better than they were at the beginning. And the reason Dr. Collins is here today is to tell us, hopefully, that the chemo has been effective.

"We're looking for a number," she says. She is standing near my bed. When she is on her rounds, she will be flanked by several other doctors, young, diligently writing notes with tiny, almost invisible pens on equally tiny, imperceptible scraps of paper. Today she is alone.

"We don't need to get into too much in the way of details here, Robert, unless you want to. The number itself isn't too important. It's a reflection of the percentage of leukemic blasts that still remain in your system, okay? It's meant to provide us with a level of confidence that your leukemia has been eradicated. This is what we're looking for."

I'm not so perky anymore. These days have been long and slow and draining. I can't think of anything funny to say. No snappy retorts to demonstrate how brave I'm being, or how I'm concerned but, you know, not too concerned. I'm tough. Tough as nails. Instead of the funny energetic wise guy, boldly laughing in the face of danger, I have become the silent warrior nodding quietly to the good doctor.

"That's fine," I say. "I don't need the details. I'm just ready to move forward."

Dr. Collins pauses. "Well, that's the problem. You still have too many blasts in your system. You still have leukemia. I'm sorry, Robert. You're not in remission."

What?

The deal is that Dr. Collins is only supposed to bring good news. That's the way it works. I do what all my doctors and nurses tell me to do — do everything with a smile on my face if I have to, gritting my teeth if necessary, no complaints — and the good news is supposed to flow like wine. We have certain expectations, understand, and they are *not* being met with this announcement.

There are, of course, explanations. It's not backpedaling. I know she's not backpedaling. And I know that what she's telling me are things that didn't make sense to explain to me at the beginning. We're optimistic on Day One. We're so completely ready to beat this thing. Day One is not the time to hear what Dr. Collins is now patiently explaining to her dumbstruck patient.

"On average," she says, "it takes 1.3 weeks of chemotherapy to induce remission."

Induce is always the word we use when we talk about remission. Induction. *Induction-duction, what's your function?*

And because my protocol calls for seven solid days of chemo, my "seven-and-three," the statistic Dr. Collins shares with us really means that far more patients make it to remission after only one week of chemo than don't. More get it right the first time, so it's not really backpedaling at all. The odds had been in my favor.

I should yell. I should totally yell at the top of my lungs that this is complete and utter bullshit. I should rage.

What the hell kind of hospital is this? What the hell kind of protocol am I on that I'm not already in remission after a week of chemotherapy? You think taking this stuff is easy? You think it's fun? I did what you told me to do! I'm supposed to be better by now!

A rage would be good, the way tough-as-nails heroes do. Knocking over hospital equipment. A big show. I can't rip the Hickman from my chest, but I could at least make sure I'm not hooked into anything when I stand up and indignantly shout "I am *so* out of here!" I could slam the door behind me on the way out, carefully — but angrily — pulling my metal card behind me. I'd slowly walk barefoot to the elevators and punch at the "down" button until it took me to the lobby. I mean, I could really *fume* in those soft lobby chairs.

I don't have a car, or money for a taxi, or anywhere to go, really, and there's no way my little buddy could fit into our getaway ride, but I could march right down to the front door and ... and ... *fuck.*

I should be so angry, but I'm not. I'm not even sad. I remember writing ominous journal entries to myself, knowing full well that my words were a scary foreshadowing of something bad just over the horizon. I should have hurriedly walked up the Spine at Lancaster University to visit a doctor at the first sign of my ridiculously obvious symptoms. Instead, I sat around and did nothing for five days. Five fucking days — with a disease that attacks with lightning speed — procrastinating, too afraid to do anything except make excuses and pretend that nothing was wrong. And *that* delay led to further unexpected delays getting here. This is my responsibility. This is all on me. Yelling at Dr. Collins won't help to get me into remission any sooner. It won't fix the mistakes I made in England.

"What does this mean?" I ask. "What's next?"

I think I already know. My sister had a blood test last week. It's a very precise test that measures six specific factors to determine whether her bone marrow and my bone marrow are identical. Siblings sometimes are. They're the best bet for a bone marrow transplant. Except — much to Laura's chagrin, apologies after apologies — she didn't match. We're still searching the registry for a better match, just in case. At least for now, I'm pretty sure that we've only got one available option for treatment.

"Same protocol as before," Dr. Collins says, "with one small difference: we're going to reverse the order. We want to hit your leukemia hard while it's on the run. We'll start both the daunorubicin and ara-C at the same time, the stronger combination at the beginning instead of the end. It's still 7+3 only this time we'll hit you harder at the start."

"Just one more week, then?"

"Yes. Same as before."

It's not as if I have a choice. This isn't really a question-and-answer session with Dr. Collins to determine what other options are available to me. There's nothing any of us can do but listen to her advice. I should have stood up last month and walked to the campus infirmary when I'd had the chance instead of thinking of clever ways to test my leg for bruising. It's a little late for regrets, isn't it?

"When do we start," I ask.

"Now. Right now. Immediately. I've already asked Cindy to start your chemo just as soon as I've finished talking with you and your mother. We need to start now."

Mom's hand is squeezing mine. Tight. I might be squeezing back just as hard. Can't be certain. I look to my right and all I can think to do is smile weakly and shrug my shoulders. She squeezes my hand once more, trying her best to not cry.

Here we go again.

CHAPTER 18

I've started to notice other patients when I go on my daily walks around the floor. There is no confusing those of us pulling our carts and chemo with visitors. Aside from the obvious rolling carts we tend to bring with us, most patients shuffle along without purpose. We're not walking with our heads up, alert, scanning the numbers outside the closed doors. We're just moving along, trying to help our legs remember what it's like to walk, one foot in front of the other until we complete the loop back to our rooms.

There isn't much in the way of small talk. I'm not here to make friends, nor do I feel much like engaging in hospitalized variations of your typical hallway conversations.

"Hi, there! How's it going?"

"*Lousy*. I've got cancer. Thanks for asking, asshole!"

New visitors will linger outside my door when I return. Sometimes it's a pack of white coats. Fresh new faces, young, earnest, ready to learn. Sometimes it will be another friend or old family member coming to visit for the first time, as the news of my "condition" (*always whispered, always quiet, when we talk in quotes about my "condition")* expands through ever-expanding circles of acquaintances.

Sometimes people are waiting for me, but quite often they are there for the woman next door. She is in the first room from the desk, the closest room. She is even closer to everything than I am. Our two doors are adjacent. The hospital is almost like an apartment complex, with entrances to rooms paired as they move down the hallway. I don't know much about this woman other than her name — Susan — and that knowledge was only glimmered from overheard conversations.

I've just come back from a slow walk. A handful of people were lingering outside my door when I'd left, and they're still here, staring at their shoes, shuffling from one foot to the other. It is a silent, uncomfortable dance. Cindy is waiting for me inside. We've got another test to do, or temperatures to take, or food to ignore, or some important something that's just like all the other somethings we've been doing for weeks.

I'm curious about the woman next door. I've never seen her before, not when I'm trying to get some exercise, or even when I'm being wheeled from one end of the hospital to the next for different tests.

"Do you know the woman over there?" I ask, nodding toward the wall that separates our two rooms.

"You mean Susan? Of course. What about her?"

"I'm just curious."

"About what?"

"I mean, you don't have to tell me if you're not supposed to, you know, or whatever, but I was kind of wondering what kind of cancer she has, you know, because I don't think I've ever seen her before."

"She doesn't have cancer," Cindy tells me. "She's in a coma."

Susan is in her mid-thirties. Cindy shares that she'd been in a pretty bad accident several months ago. She doesn't appear to respond to anything — light, noise, proximity of family members, anything. I assume she must be getting her "food" the same way that I am, nutrients from a bag, dripping into a tube. It doesn't sound like she's in critical condition; there's a separate ward for that. She still needs a great deal of personalized care from a crack nursing staff who can pay attention to details, but she's not hanging by a thread.

My bed faces the wall that separates our two rooms. It's easy to stare at it when I'm lying in bed, easy to stare at that wall and just let the view blur and fade to black.

I've been getting more fevers lately. Bad ones. They spike pretty high: 104, 105, 106, something like that. One minute I will be so unbearably hot that Mom and Cindy will constantly replace ice cold towels on my chest and forehead. They soak white hand towels in a wide bowl filled with ice. Then the fever will swing and I'll be so cold that my body shakes. I'm freezing. Cindy rushes out to get a pile of hot blankets. I'm curled in a fetal position, shaking uncontrollably, teeth literally chattering. I never knew that was really a thing. I can't stop my teeth from chattering. I can't do anything about any of it. Cindy stacks the hot blankets three or four high on top of me before leaving again to get the only thing that seems to help anymore: Demerol.

She comes back with a needle. She swipes alcohol across an open port on my Hickman with one hand, then swiftly plunges the

Demerol into my bloodstream. It doesn't take long before my muscles relax and the chills go away.

Everything gets fuzzy. I stretch out my legs and stare at the wall. My face is starting to get numb. I try not to think about things too much. If I start thinking about the details then I'll be able to find all sorts of things to worry about. The fevers are more than a little scary. They're not terrible, not really, but they keep coming back, and they do worse things to my body than the nausea. Where are they coming from? When will they stop? What if there's an infection someplace bad, like my lungs, or my brain?

See? See. This is *exactly* why I need to stop thinking about everything so much. What ifs and imagined worst-case scenarios don't help at all.

The Demerol cuts the edge. I'm blinking in super slow motion, like a super slow-motion superhero. My eyes are ballistic. Eyelids shut with a slam. Everything goes dark. *Bam*!

Open again. The wall between our rooms is still there. My feet poke out from underneath a pile of blankets. You can't handle this, these eyelids of super-slowness. They slam shut again. They are heavy. I'm just blinking, but it's slower and more heroic than anything you can imagine.

My eyes sweep open, running a quick status check. Lines are still connected, blood is still pumping, stomach is neither happy nor unhappy. Fever is probably feverish, still, but I'm okay. All systems check out okay. I'm not great, but not terrible, either. It could be worse.

This is what my Grandpa Soder — Mom's dad — always used to say. Ask him about anything. Ask him about the stock market, the Mariners, weather in Portland, or his well-done steak dinner. *How was the steak, Grandpa? How have you been?*

"Could be better, could be worse."

Of course it could be better! That's an easy answer: let's go back in time six weeks or eight weeks or something and wave a magic wand so I never had leukemia. But that's not very likely. That's not realistic. We've got to play with the hand we've been dealt. And it could be so much worse, too. I mean, I could be dead already. Should be dead, maybe.

So let's not go there. Let's not think about it being that much worse. Today's not bad. Today is okay. But there was that one time, a week or so ago? Vomiting then was much worse than it is now. And, wow, I can't imagine spiking a temp as bad as that one a few days ago. Look at my arms and side: I'm not even bleeding anymore. *That* was bad, bleeding from my Hickman. I don't want to push the logical inconsistencies with this: that my worst days couldn't *all* be in the past.

I'm not losing any limbs to the cancer, which would easily be much worse than what I'm experiencing. Leukemia doesn't spread, or metastasize, or need to be operated out. I don't want to go under the knife. What if I needed to have my leg amputated just below the knee? I've seen other patients with other cancers during our walks. I feel bad. I feel bad that their cancer is so much more visible than mine. Tumors that need to be cut out, body parts to be discarded.

I might still be in England, far from home, with no visitors coming in and out every day. Mom told me that Pan Am had the right to refuse the second flight, because of my reaction to blood before getting on the first. She'd been working out different angles while I'd slept in a London hospital. Through friends of friends at Boeing with connections to the military she'd found a backup plan for us: some kind of trans-Atlantic military transport to get me home in case Pan Am had balked.

But even that could have fallen through. What then? The protocol would have been the same, I'm sure, and the hospitals in London would be top-notch, but I'd still be a stranger in a strange land, wishing I was somewhere else. No good could come of two weeks of chemotherapy working against a lonely, homesick heart.

Cindy and Anne might not have cared about me as much as they do. They could have been crisp and professional and maybe a little cool. Distant. I might have had different nurses altogether.

There are so many ways it could have been different. So many countless ways it could have been worse. I stare through the dark at Susan's wall and I'm mostly just sad. None of what I'm going through seems all bad compared to being on the other side of that wall.

CHAPTER 19

The additional week of chemo, frontloaded with the nastier, stronger ara-c, turns what had been a minor nuisance into something more. More constant, more ever-present, this pit in my stomach. The taste, too. God. I can't get rid of it, even with all the mints Mom brings for me to devour. It's internal. The taste comes from inside somewhere, and mints do nothing for it.

You can emulate what my chemo tastes like, short term, by getting your key chain. Pick a key, any key. House, car, bike lock, whatever. Something nice and good and metallic and suck on it for a few minutes. Taste it. Enjoy the taste for a few minutes only but, please, do not drink a tall cold glass of milk. We have already learned that certain foods and tastes don't mix all that well with that delicious metallic taste of chemo.

My stomach isn't very happy with me. It doesn't take much anymore. Just the smell of somebody else's food moving past my door, just a hint of a smell of something edible is enough to send me racing to the bathroom.

I've moved well past the stage of actually thinking it's kind of cool to just puke all the time. You know, strange things happening to your body, marveling at the way it reacts to new situations and new environments? I'm vomiting for no reason at all. Whoop-de-fucking-do. The novelty has worn off. The fact that my body is reacting to chemo is no longer gee-whiz cool. It's just shitty, now, all the time, a necessary condition on the road to remission.

I don't bring it up. I don't ask for any drugs or anything. But I am past the point of keeping up a brave face all the time, shiny happy patient, pretending like the stomach flip-flops and constant kneeling visits to the toilet don't bother me. It is remarkable what can happen when you tell the people who care about you how you're feeling.

"You know, Robert," Cindy says one afternoon, "we can try to do something about the nausea."

"Stop my chemo?" I ask. No harm in asking.

She chuckles. "No. Not that. We can give you medical marijuana. It helps ease things for some people. It just kind of evens out your stomach. It can help you to feel like you don't have to throw up all the time."

I'm not at all comfortable with Cindy's suggestion.

It's not like I'm embarrassed about it, but my doctors and nurses are always so matter-of-fact. I don't want to say no, because I'm sure Cindy wouldn't suggest it if they didn't think it was a good idea, I just don't like it at all.

I've seen patients downstairs. They stand together in the rising sun, wearing bathrobes or pajamas or hospital-issued gowns, just beyond the sliding glass doors leading outdoors. They need their cigarettes. They need their morning nicotine fix. Some I've even seen back upstairs, here on the cancer ward with me. I know that it's a lifetime of smoking that creates those kinds of habits, not just a joint or two, but the last thing I want to do is join that parade of frowning faces outside the main entrance, smoking not so much because I want to, but because I have to.

Doctor's orders, I will tell them as I smoke pot from my wheelchair. *Honest.*

"Umm ... I'm sorry, Cindy, but I don't smoke. I don't much feel like starting, either. Is there anything else?"

Spontaneous laughter. A smile as warm as the sun.

"Oh, it's not like that," she says. "It's a marijuana *pill*. Synthetic. We'll give you a pill."

I'm both optimistic and skeptical about this new pill. I still don't understand how marijuana — even in a synthetic pill-like form — is going to help with the nausea.

"It's something we give to patients all the time," Cindy says. "It's not like you'll get high or anything, if that's what you mean, but it helps take the edge off. I don't know how else to explain it. I can get you more information if you'd like."

I don't think I've yet gone against a recommendation from Cindy, Anne, Dr. Collins. Anyone involved with my treatment, really. I'll ask plenty of questions. I will try to gather as much data about a new procedure, or a new medicine, trying to understand symptoms and side effects and everything, but I've never said "no." I trust their judgment. Anything to help with my nausea at this point must be a good thing.

And so I try it. Tiny pills that I drink with a room temperature glass of apple juice. I'm not sure if it works at first. It seems to work. It almost immediately seems to work. At least I think it does. I can't really tell.

My stomach begins to relax. I don't feel quite so rough, quite so ready to run to the bathroom if a milk commercial comes on the TV, or somebody walks past my room with a bag of fast food. So I'm thinking it must be working, right, because the badness is less bad? That's good.

The odd thing is that after a few hours or so I find myself getting hungry. I mean, I am so completely *not* hungry that this is a little surprising. I haven't had anything resembling an appetite for weeks now. My "meals" still come exclusively from the big bag of TPN dripping into my catheter. My mouth still tastes like metal. I know I'm not hungry, but I can't help it.

I don't even want to *think* about food, but I'm feeling like a cheeseburger would taste great right now. A Kidd Valley burger with a side of fries and a strawberry shake. Maybe onion rings, too. I'm fucking famished. What the hell?

I could call Dad or Jane, and I bet they'd bring me something when they come to visit. *Mmm.* I want to dip those onion rings in tartar sauce! So delicious. I can practically taste the food, it's been so long, my imagination suddenly working overdrive.

Reality jolts. Another sensation — more familiar, more easily recognized — interrupts my thoughts. This is what the pills were supposed to prevent. I'm scrambling to get out of bed to make it to my bathroom in time.

Good afternoon, Mr. Toilet. Looks like these medical marijuana pills didn't work after all.

* * *

We try again. We try several times over the course of several days. I'm really trying to pay attention, to notice how everything feels, both before and after. The frustrating thing is that it always seems like it's working at first, but then it almost always goes bad after a few hours. I'm always getting hungry.

And then it dawns on me: although I never smoked pot in college, I was more than familiar with some of the after-effects. The guys down the hall would come pounding on doors, just shy of two o'clock in the morning. *My dudes! Domino's is closing soon. Does anybody wanna get a pizza? Anyone? Like an extra-large pepperoni or something?*

Funny stuff. Hilarious. These are the unexpected consequences of a pill that I will no longer be taking, even though it turns out that they were working fine all along. It wasn't that I was ever truly hungry at all. Even with medical marijuana, it was the *munchies* that were killing me.

CHAPTER 20

Everything has been low, okay, almost from day one: overall blood counts, platelets, polys (or neutrophils), red blood cells, white blood cells, weight, energy, hair follicles, whatever. You name it, I didn't have enough of it. Nature of the beast.

We're getting technical, though, learning new words all the time. This isn't just throwing all the medicine available at me hoping some of it sticks. There is real science involved here, culled from decades of research. Details matter. Precision matters. That's why we notice when certain things change, when certain thresholds are crossed. It's not an obvious one, at least not to me, initially, but this line clearly marks a difference in how we'll need to approach my treatment. We're all about numbers these days, watching the steady drop of so many different counts. We watch my polys closely. They're a leading indicator. When they'd dropped low enough, earlier in my first exhausting week of chemotherapy, Dr. Collins had given me a new word to describe things: *Neutropenia.*

I had become neutropenic. My counts were too low. A colored sign had been placed outside my door, probably red, to remind all visitors (and hospital staff) that they would need to take precautions once they entered my room. When I'm neutropenic, my body will struggle that much more to fight infections. Without enough neutrophils, there's little my body can do to fend for itself. And we know that I'm not capable of producing any new neutrophils. There's only one direction that count has been able to go and it sure isn't up – at least not until after I manage to get in remission.

It also makes sense that I've been getting fevers. They arrive out of nowhere, though, with increasing frequency and strength. They are very mysterious. Very crafty. My doctors haven't yet tracked down the source, but they still make sense. This is my body behaving the way it should when the numbers are what they are.

See, that's the thing now. I'm not *just* neutropenic anymore. My extra week of chemo, especially those first three days, did a real number on my numbers. Whatever straggling triple-digit poly count I had going into that week was quickly eradicated. I've bottomed out. I quite literally have nothing left: my blood counts are at zero. Is there a good term for that? *Superneutropenic?*

Every return fever, now, is cause for more concern. This is why I'm hooked up to so many different antibiotics, why Cindy and Anne spend so much extra time in my room. They're constantly swapping out meds, monitoring my temp, trying to head things off before they get bad. Everything takes on a greater sense of urgency when your immune system has stopped working.

My doctors have to be more aggressive in their search for what's been causing all of my fevers. They can't just appear on their own, out of nowhere, out of thin air. They're symptomatic of something else: one or more infections, somewhere. Fevers have to have a source. They have to originate from somewhere inside my body. *But where?* There are no obvious answers.

We've kept my Hickman clean. There are no festering sores or oozing pus around the entry site. When I take two deep breaths with a cold stethoscope on my chest, then two more with the stethoscope on my back, my lungs sound clean and clear. We've started scheduling multiple X-rays to validate that there are no infections in my lungs.

I should expect these fevers, right, with my superneutropenia and all, but while it's okay to *expect* them, Dr. Collins absolutely will not *tolerate* them. Unless I'm able to magically stop them on my own — *which I can't, no matter how hard I try* — then she will continue to search relentlessly for the source. It's not good enough to just keep on keeping on.

Demerol helps, almost instantaneously, with my convulsive chills. Tylenol manages to ease my throbbing headaches and to reduce my sky-high temps. Together, they form an effective one-two punch against my fevers, but they don't do anything about eliminating the source. That's what my doctors are after. That's the mystery we want to solve.

* * *

We're trying something new. Dr. Collins has prescribed a new drug, designed to take care of one of the many possible sources of my fevers. The drug is called amphotericin. Apparently, it's ridiculously strong. There are lots of potentially negative side effects, but the working theory is that this might take care of my fevers by taking out the source.

"Funny thing," Anne explains to me the first night. She's going to be giving me my first dose. "You'll think it's really funny, Robert."

"What?" *Wheel of Fortune* has just wrapped up, and *Jeopardy* is about to start. Anne had waited until the commercial break between the shows before beginning to prep me for my new drug. I've never watched either these TV shows at home, or at Carleton, but here I'm a captive audience. There's little else to do. I have come to absolutely love the marketing genius behind scheduling these two shows back-to-back. Lowbrow to highbrow. I'm not even ashamed to admit that I'm hooked. They're as good an addiction as any to have while I'm still in the hospital.

"The amphotericin — *ampho* — has some side effects. I'm sure Dr. Collins has told you this already."

I just stare at Anne. I'm sure Dr. Collins did, too, but I can't remember any of it.

"We need to prep you, first, before you get the ampho. We need to mitigate those side effects."

"And?" I love Anne's company, I really do. But the commercials are wrapping up, and this is looking like it might cut into my very important television time. How can I prove how much smarter I am than the *Jeopardy* contestants if we're busy talking about medicine?

She smiles patiently. "One of the side effects, Mr. Brown, is that you might spike some pretty high temps."

"I've been getting high temperatures for days," I whine. "I don't want more!"

"I know. This is all about treating infections, though, not fevers. Dr. Collins wants to make sure you don't have an infection, somewhere, that's ultimately been *causing* your fevers. We all do, Robert. This should help."

"Okay," I say. I'm trying to focus on our discussion. "So this amphotericin will help fight a possible infection that's causing my fevers, but in doing so it might give me a fever?"

"Most likely, yes." She smiles again. "And how do we manage those fevers? With Tylenol aaaand…?"

"Seriously?"

She doesn't need to answer. We will be proactively giving me the things that have had the best impact on keeping my fevers down, because the new drug that we want to use to eliminate those same fevers has a side effect that could include, you know, a fucking fever.

"What's first?" I ask.

"Tylenol, first, followed by Demerol. Same as usual."

Those two alone are quite the cocktail, let alone the addition a bit later of the amphotericin. Anne and I will watch *Jeopardy* together repeatedly. The timing of my ampho doses needs to be consistent in order for it to be most effective. Same time every night.

She starts getting ready when Wheel of Fortune is winding down, setting out needles, writing down a few notes for the overnight staff. I get my Tylenol down as soon as Jeopardy starts. She pushes the Demerol into my Hickman. The edges start to smooth down. Time slows. My face gets fuzzy. Anne and I wait until the first commercial break. She sits lightly on the edge of my bed, these ten or fifteen minutes of quiet time, our time, both of us trying to beat the so-serious contestants on the TV.

Time crawls. I forget the question. The answer, I mean. You're supposed to answer Alex Trebek's question with a question, right? Confusion and fatigue settle in. Anne asks if I'm ready. I think I probably nod, or shrug, or just close my eyes, still trying to find words that mean anything.

She plunges the ampho. It's warm. It is quite the mix. I try to hold on, try to stay awake until Final Jeopardy. It's a futile struggle, so I just let go.

* * *

Dr. Collins is thoughtful. She stands next to my bed, eyes raised to the ceiling, thinking about the question I've just asked her. See, I don't know what I don't know, and I've asked her to help me understand. I'd asked Dr. Gorst a similar question, barely a few weeks ago now. *What are my odds?*

I'd wanted something concrete. Numbers are facts. They are real. They have weight. You can lash yourself to them to help weather the storm. I remember him telling me that leukemia had an 80% survival rate. I did not push back. I never asked for clarification. *Eighty percent of what? Survival for how long? Is this for childhood leukemias, or the kind that I have?*

It's not that I don't believe those numbers, not exactly, I'm just wondering if he told me what he thought a stupid, scared American college student needed to hear. That's why I've asked Dr. Collins. She'll be straight with me. She always is.

"I'm going to be completely honest with you, Robert," she finally says. She makes eye contact. She takes a step closer, almost reaching out to touch my shoulder. She's a good doctor, my good doctor. "You're asking me what I think your chances of survival are, right?"

I nod. Cindy had been here earlier to give me some Demerol. Stupid fevers. The Demerol helps with the chills, of course, as it always does, but it also always makes everything fuzzy. I rub my face with my right hand, starting at my forehead, lingering at the bridge of my nose before continuing a slow swipe down to my chin. I'm not sure if I can feel anything.

"You might hear different numbers, depending on who you talk to," Dr. Collins continues. "There's a fair amount of ongoing debate, especially with your M3 subtype. And you already know that most AML patients are typically much older than you. That's why I want you to understand that the numbers, the charts, they're all irrelevant. High-level statistics don't matter, Robert.

"Your odds aren't ten percent, or twenty, or even fifty. You either survive or you don't. Period. You are *alive* today! Such a wonderful thing! That means your *personal* chances of survival, the only ones that matter, right now, this moment, are at one hundred percent. With each new day under your belt it's the same story. One day at a time, Robert, you have a hundred percent chance.

"Does that make sense? Does that help?"

I nod again. I still can't feel my face, so I check once more to make sure it's there.

✳ ✳ ✳

It's a repeat. My life is on repeat. Stupid daily tests and regular antibiotics to fight stupid fucking fevers that I'm only getting because of what my doctors have done to me. It feels like the same thing every day. Blood counts are gone. Immune system is gone. Appetite is so long gone I can't imagine that I've ever wanted to eat solid food. Michele comes in most days with her scale-on-wheels and those numbers continue to drop, too. I'm wasting away. I'm down into the 150's for the first time since, what, middle school? Freshman year?

At least my second week of chemo is finally done!

In a repeat of an identical discussion a little more than a week ago — *has it already been that long?* — we've scheduled yet another bone marrow biopsy. It'll be my third one in about a month. Lucky me. And Dr. Collins tells all of us, again, that this will be the definitive test. This will be the one that answers with striking clarity the question that's been on all of our minds recently. *Am I in remission?*

And when the results come back only a short while later, I'd expected I'd greet the good news with much fanfare and hoopla. I've been waiting so long for any kind of good news that I'd thought I'd have the energy to jump up and hug Dr. Collins. There would be singing and dancing! Dr. Collins in some cheesy musical routine with the other attending physicians as her backup dancers, jazz hands and fancy footwork. There'd be laughter and cheering and wondrous joy at the news. Disco balls drop down from the ceiling tiles, confetti explodes from cannons in the corners of my room! There's a standing ovation thundering from the halls, all the other patients, their families, the entire hospital, cars honking in the parking lot, all united in their chanting cheers.

Robert! Remission! Robert! Remission!

Don't get me wrong. It is great, finally, that the results of this most recent bone marrow biopsy show that the second week of chemo worked. It's great to be in remission. Great with a capital "G" and a Tony the Tiger drawl! If the additional week of chemotherapy hadn't sent my leukemia packing, I don't know what we would have done. A third week of chemo? Doubt I could have survived it. A bone marrow transplant? With no donor lined up, and no perfect match for me anyway, even if we could have coordinated everything, found somebody willing to donate their not-quite-right-for-me-marrow, timed it right, odds are I'd likely end up rejecting the transplant anyway. *Graft-Versus-Host Disease*, is what they call that, when the new bone marrow (*graft*) takes a look around at my body (*host*) and says "this isn't right" before attacking what it perceives to be a foreign body. Except it's not something foreign. It's me. It's my body that's being rejected by the very thing that's supposed to save it.

No chance for more chemotherapy and no viable transplant options? *No, thank you.* Remission is exactly where I want to be. A week or so earlier I'd probably do a little jig, you know, my funky little eighties dance where I don't actually lift my bare feet from the floor, just plant them close together, my upper body doing most of the moving, trying to pay attention to the back beat, hands in these loose fists. It works well for me, because it's a low energy kind of dance style. I mean, you're gonna break a sweat if you keep at it for a couple of hours — or if the DJ decides to mix up the techno with some old school *Rock Lobster*, or even older school *Twist and Shout*, both songs forcing you to get down, down, down, close to the floor, then up, up, up again — but you're not going to be sucking wind after only a few minutes, either. It's a good hospital room dance. You can wear your pajamas for a dance like that. Your dangling Hickman catheter won't get tangled.

A week ago, even, had I learned that I'd gone into remission, I would have done that dance, still tethered to my little buddy. We would have stood in place together, my bag-holding friend and I, and we would have done our Cabbage Patch, or Churn the Butter, or whatever you call it when you're all happy about everything and dance moves are limited. *Go Robert, go Robert, go!*

But now? Now it's fever this, fever that, practically every minute of every day. I'm going to radiology regularly, taking amphotericin daily (*which really fucks me up*), ramping up the frequency of my blood tests. I can't remember the last time I've eaten, which brings up a whole different set of concerns. I'm not miserable, not really, but I'm not far from it. This is a grind. I had no idea it would take this long, and even though remission is absolutely essential to my long-term health, I'm still hanging on by a thread.

There is simply no time to celebrate and it feels premature to do a victory dance. I'm not out of the woods yet. There is still much work to be done.

CHAPTER 21

Laura stops by to visit after donating platelets. She breezes into my room. I'm always happy to see her, and not just because her platelets do a great job of bumping up my counts. Between her and Mom's donations, I continue to get the best boosts to my blood counts. Family platelets are far better for me.

There's usually not much to tell about the whole process. Laura spends a couple of hours at the blood center before driving to the hospital for a quick visit. The platelets arrive shortly after she does. They arrive by ambulance.

"Hey," she says. "I've got to tell you something. Kinda funny. Kinda gross."

"Yeah? What's that?"

She laughs, pulls her chair up closer to my bed. "I'm at the blood center, you know, hooked up to the machine."

That's how you get the platelets. I've never actually seen the machine, just heard it described many times before. You're sitting down, one arm extended, needles and tubes. Because you're only there to donate a very specific part of your blood, not whole blood, the tubes lead first to a machine. It's called a "spinning machine."

Different components of blood have different weights, different densities. The tube extracts a certain amount of whole blood before the machine fires up. The spinning inside the machine causes the blood to separate. There's another tube attached somewhere that the platelets begin to separate, and a small plastic bag is slowly filled. What doesn't go into the bag for me goes back into my sister's body. She gets all her non-platelet blood back.

Once, when Mom was donating platelets, the blood bank hadn't spun off enough of her blood from the platelets. The mix wasn't quite as pure as it could have been, and I ended up having a reaction. Red spots on my arms and legs, an almost immediate rash, a good, high temperature spike, much like what had happened in England. After that, the blood bank took extra care to make sure that the platelets were well-spun.

Blood to machine. Spin. Separate. Blood back to body. More blood to machine. Spin again. Separate again. Return again. This continues for an hour or so, until the smaller bag has been filled.

"Usually I just read when it's spinning," Laura says. "But I happened to glance at the machine, once, when I'd turned the pages. There was something different about my blood this time. Not your platelets. Those looked fine. My blood was collecting there in the machine and it looked wrong somehow. I asked one of the nurses for help."

"What was wrong?" I ask.

"Patience!" she laughs, reaching across to slap my leg. "The nurse came over and looked at my machine. She tapped it a couple of times. I'm not sure how to describe it, but there was this additional layer — some kind of clear liquid — that I've never seen before. 'Eat lunch recently?' the nurse asked. 'McDonald's? Burger King?'

"No…"

Laura nods. "It was Jack in the Box. I was running late for the appointment, so I just grabbed a cheeseburger and rings from the drive through. You know how she knew? All the fat in my lunch was getting collected, too. It was still in my blood. You should have seen it. All that cheese and grease. It was totally like the grease jar under the sink. Disgusting!"

"Yum! Does that mean I'll be getting to enjoy your cheeseburger with my platelets?"

She laughs. "Nope. I got it right back after the platelets were spun out. I asked if they could spin the fat out, too, but they wouldn't, or couldn't, so I got it right back."

She shudders, briefly, her whole body shivering once, like she's really cold, or she's just swallowed a gulp of the wrong drink from the wrong plastic cup at a crowded party, Jägermeister instead of Amstel Light. She sticks out her tongue. "If I never eat fast food again," she says, "it will be too soon."

CHAPTER 22

S eems like I've got an appointment in radiology every day now. I'm sure that there are any number of conversations that take place between Dr. Collins and my parents, details that aren't exactly hidden from me, but that are filtered down, summarized, presented to me on a need-to-know basis. My fevers are persistent. The ampho is probably working. I mean, it has to be working, even though the fevers haven't stopped, which means that probably my fevers had more than one source and only one of those sources has been dealt with.

Meanwhile, we're still searching for root causes. There's nothing obvious, nothing external, so I make several visits to the radiology department. My doctors want to take a peek inside. Just a peek. There must be something amiss, and hopefully the X-rays will help solve the mystery.

When it's getting close to the time to head down, an orderly brings a wheelchair to my room. It's almost always a tentative knock on my door. Dad follows alongside for the first couple of trips, helping steer my "little buddy," a steady hand on my shoulder, remembering the many twists and turns through wide, mostly empty hallways. After a while he takes over. When the orderlies arrive, Dad tells them that he can take it from here. They don't protest much, hurrying back to wherever it is that orderlies congregate.

We're on our way out when we pass a larger-than-usual crowd in front of Susan's room. Red, yellow, and blue streamers have been taped outside her door. A cluster of helium-free balloons hang listlessly in the corners. Unfamiliar faces wait quietly outside, whispering, some holding brightly-wrapped presents. They move out of our way. They line up against the wall to my right, smiling, nodding, waving courteously.

"What's the occasion?" I ask.

A middle-aged man answers. He looks vaguely familiar. Hair thinning at the top, closely cropped, turning silvery-gray at the sides. Must be her father. He makes eye contact, which is nice, because I've learned that usually people in wheelchairs make other people uncomfortable.

"It's Susan's birthday," he says. "We're having a party. You're more than welcome to stop by later, if you want. If you can. We have plenty of cake. Please stop by later. Help yourself."

"Thanks. Will do. We're just heading out for some X-rays."

"Good luck," he says. "See you when you get back."

* * *

We're walking to radiology together, me and my dad. He's really doing the walking for the both of us, pushing me along these empty corridors, but I like to think that I'm doing something other than sitting in this wheelchair.

I don't ask my parents too many questions. It probably doesn't even dawn on me that I should ask them how they're feeling. We're in survival mode. We don't think. We just do. We are this action-oriented family, taking me to my various appointments, or holding my hand while I sleep, or bringing packets of cards and letters that were sent to the house instead of the hospital. There's not much to discuss, I guess, when we all know that as bad as it gets, it's all part of the price. Daily trips to radiology — as exhausting as they can be — are required.

I keep my thoughts to myself on this trip, wondering what my Action Family would do if it was me in Susan's room. What if I was in a coma? Would I even be aware of it? Would I be in some kind of constant dream state, or would the screen be like snow after midnight, when the local channels have gone off the air? Would my parents need to make a decision for me? About me? Would they need to decide together?

They've been divorced almost my entire life and have always done an admirable job of remaining civil towards one another, even during a particularly difficult stretch of custody-wrangling when I was eleven. I don't remember that period of my life very well. My sister does. She has a very good memory. She'll tell both of our parents, later, that they need to stop worrying about not being in the same room together when they visit me, to not make the important part of the hospital visit the fact that one has to suddenly leave as soon as the other arrives. But how do you set apart twenty years of being apart? How do you simply come together in a snap of your fingers like that?

What if I was in a coma? I'd be alive, right, but not really. My hands wouldn't even twitch when Mom held them in hers. My face is a blank, unmoving slate. You hope, of course, that everything you do or say registers somewhere underneath the surface, but how long does that keep you going? Weeks? Months? Could it be years? How long do you continue to watch your child do nothing, say nothing, respond to nothing? How do you even imagine a point where you need to consider the possibility that you maybe need to make this very important decision for your child?

She's in her mid-thirties, Susan. She's not a child, but she's still their child, and she's completely, totally, dependent on the decisions made by her parents. Does she even know it's her birthday? Does she even know about the balloons and the streamers and the presents?

* * *

My appointment takes a couple of hours. Too much of that time is spent waiting in the cold hallway outside the waiting room, always as far away from other sick patients as possible. We'd wrapped a lightweight blanket around my shoulders to keep me warm.

When they'd finally made time to bring me in, it turns out we needed more X-rays than normal. Maybe Dr. Collins had ordered some additional shots, or maybe the technician saw something interesting and wanted to get more detail, or maybe they just screwed up the whole thing and didn't bother to tell me that they needed to do things over. Whatever the case, there was a lot of standing and turning and holding my breath, and *turn again, please, hold still, please*, and, as I moved to sit back down, *we're not quite done yet, please.* I'm exhausted.

After the elevator returns us to my floor, I ask Dad to leave the wheelchair at the main desk. I need to keep using my legs. There are so few opportunities, what with everybody wanting me to stay in my room as much as possible ever since I became neutropenic. My legs are already skinnier and weaker than they've ever been. Even though I don't really want to walk, I know that I should. It's only ten feet or so from the desk to my door. At least it's something.

The crowd outside Susan's room has left. It is quiet. Streamers and balloons still run along the door frame, a swirl of primary colors. I'd forgotten about her birthday party. Her door is open, but not by much. I turn to look at Dad.

"Whaddya think?" I ask. "Think it's okay to go in?"

"Seems pretty quiet," he says.

"I'll just knock. Her dad said to stop by, right? I can just knock and see."

There's no response, so I knock louder. Then: two voices, male and female, both at the same time, "come in, come in." The curtains are drawn and the lights are off, but there's still enough daylight to see into the room. I motion for Dad to follow. Susan's parents are sitting together in the chairs lined against the windows on the opposite side of the room. They stand as we enter, walking quietly over to shake hands and introduce themselves.

"I'm sorry," I say, smiling underneath my surgical mask, keeping my hands to my side. "Infections, you know. I have to be careful."

Dad does the hand-shaking for both of us. He stands next to me, his left hand on my back, introductions with his right. Even though I'm pretty sure he's met Susan's parents before, he does the name thing again, for my sake.

Susan's room is exactly like mine. I mean, of course I don't have all the birthday decorations, a half-eaten chocolate cake with chocolate frosting in the recessed space underneath the TV set, a matching set of red plastic plates, cups, napkins and forks waiting for guests to serve themselves. And it's backwards. It's right-ways for her and her parents but it's backwards for me, a mirror image, sinks and doors and windows in places that make sense for others, but not for me. It's like a Bizarro World version, but without all the rough angles and frustrated super villains.

I gravitate to the cards and letters on her bulletin boards. I'm a complete sucker when it comes to reading what other people have written. When I was seventeen or eighteen, visiting Dad and Jane in Long Beach when they'd moved to California for a few years, we visited the famed La Brea Tar Pits. Dinosaur bones, yeah, mud, concrete, tar, whatever the hell they sunk in. You can read about it. Rent the audio tape and listen to the droning narration as you look around, unable to find anything exciting or dramatic about the slow deaths of creatures that had lived hundreds of thousands of years ago. It's historic, and epic, just not my cup of tea.

But what's this? In the middle of an expansive hallway, there, behind numerous glass display cases, local schoolchildren had written (and sometimes illustrated) letters of thanks. This was something I could get excited about. Big pieces of white paper, with big grade school handwriting that invariably started largest on the left of the page, then scrunched smaller and smaller the closer it got to the edge. No sense worrying about punctuation, spelling, or capitalization. None of that really mattered. Every letter was this stunning display of genuine thanks. You could feel the shimmering emotion behind the crayon drawings of T-Rexes and Stegosauruses and Pterodactyls.

Dad and Jane were surprised, later, when they asked what I'd liked best about the Tar Pits and I launched into this detailed description of David Ortega's heartfelt letter, Jeremy's incredibly lifelike drawings, and Beth! Walker's! Prolific! Exclamation! Points! They were the only things in the whole place that actually felt *alive*, the only things that captured my interest.

I move to Susan's bulletin boards, first, instead of to her bed, partly because I'm drawn to what other people write, always have been, curious what her loved ones would write to her, but also because it's the farthest point in the room from her. Truth is that I'm instantly awkward, suddenly ashamed that I've been in the hospital for a month and this is the first time I've ever visited. And I'm not even visiting, not really, I'm just answering an invite from her father by glomming onto the wall that separates our two rooms.

Not that I'm about to walk up and down the halls — knocking on everybody's door, checking in, checking up — but she's literally right next door. I can't leave my room without walking past hers.

"But I'm sick," I tell myself.

You're just lying around half the time anyway, I answer back.

"But I'm here to get better, not socialize..."

Common courtesy, asshole. Her parents are going through a lot.

"What? *My* parents are going through a lot," I say.

Now you're just being selfish.

"That's ridiculous!" I'm starting to get pretty angry with myself now.

It's always got to be about you, doesn't it?

Susan's mom interrupts my inner dialogue. I'm just staring at the bulletin board, still, and she gently touches my shoulder. "Excuse me," she says. "Did you want some cake? I'm sure Susan would like you to have some."

She sees me eyeing the multicolored rectangles of paper on the wall and must think that I've been focused on the party food that's between the two bulletin boards. "No," I say. "No thank you. I really can't eat anything."

She apologizes. There's this sadness behind her eyes. She says I'm sorry and it feels so very sad, more than it should, her hands folded together, eyes downcast.

"Do you want some for later? We could wrap some up for you."

I know I'm not going to eat it. Just thinking about it starts a minor chain reaction, from wanting to remember what moist chocolate cake tastes like — licking frosting from my fingers, washing it all down with an ice-cold glass of milk — to my empty stomach grumbling, sending a brief, heaving warning to my brain. I'm not going to eat a single bite, but I nod anyway.

"Please. Yes, please." I say.

Susan's mother had come prepared. She removes a serrated knife and a roll of Saran Wrap from a crumpled, well-used grocery bag on the floor. The knife edge is wrapped in foil. She cuts into the cake as if she's drawing a line, then a little wiggle, the smaller piece separated from the rest of the cake. She carefully balances a hefty slice on the flat of the knife, setting it onto one of the few large red plates remaining. Saran Wrap is doubled around the plate.

She tucks it in. Creases the edges, both thumbs and forefingers starting at twelve o'clock, meeting again at six.

"It's good," she says. "I made it myself."

CHAPTER 23

I t's not a game, but it should be. We should have a contest. How high do we think my temps will run today? How many times will I need some Demerol to keep my teeth from chattering uncontrollably, to help me find any kind of warmth under the stacks of hot blankets, piping hot, steaming, like a Robert pancake?

Or what about guessing the other numbers that we're constantly monitoring: my absolute dearth of any measurable blood counts? Will they be coming back today? Which ones? We'd like something. Polys would be fantastic. They would be perfect, in fact, the best line of defense against elusive infections, but we don't want to get carried away. Some of my own platelets would be cool, too. *Anything.*

Any new blood counts would be fucking outstanding. Any little blip on the chart to demonstrate that my bone marrow is waking up again — still woozy from being knocked out by the chemo, shaking off the pain, slowly, slowly finding a way to get up off the mat. Remission is meaningless until my counts come back.

Pulling my catheter is a last resort. It's the last thing any of us wants to do, but we've looked damn near everywhere and there's no stopping these fevers.

We will check one final time, another new test. It's something I'd never heard of before, a bronchoscopy. Dr. Collins wants to see if we could approach the problem from a different angle. X-rays afford a view of the inside of my body, but from the outside. They're flat. They're all black and white and shades of gray, and mistakes can be made. Of course we check from the front and the back, and from each side, me, wearily, standing and turning, turning, turning, turning, but lung infections can still hide from the technician.

The bronchoscopy gives us something much better: a view from the inside, in color, live action. Better technology, better quality images, better everything. All these improvements do not come without a price. The procedure itself is nowhere near as simple as an X-ray, which requires little more of me than simply standing and turning, over and again. It's not nearly as invasive and permanent as, say, getting my Hickman catheter.

Again, it's all relative. I am admittedly not the best with getting stuff down my throat. The chemo has made it worse. I've been making strides, though, learning how to effortlessly swallow pills while drinking juice, but I'm still not at all good with solids foods, solid anything. The prospect of a long tube snaking down my throat is pretty disconcerting. It'll be long and thin, the tube — at least two, maybe three feet long. It will pass through my open mouth and down my neck at which point the doctor will work some magic, using the tiny fiber-optic camera on the end to find an angle into my right lung. It's a flexible tube. Space age materials, I'm sure. All very high-tech.

The doctor had told me his name, earlier, and I've already forgotten it. He explained that even though the tube was flexible, all fancy and expensive, it wouldn't move on its own. It was spaghetti-like, but not spaghetti, understand? You ever do that trick? In the cafeteria at college, just goofing around, where you get a long strand of spaghetti and you swallow it halfway so part of it's just dangling out your mouth? You can bend over the table and wiggle it around by moving your head; because the other half is in your body, it's not going anywhere. Half the table says "gross" while the other half laughs, so instead of just swallowing it you pull it back out.

The bronchoscopy doctor is navigating this tube up and down my neck, in and out of my lungs, cameras rolling. This is the price we need to pay for higher quality images — the best quality images — of my lungs. *Infections? You there? We'll find you if you are.*

I'm breathing. I am trying to breathe.

Relax, Robert. Just. Just. *Relax.*

It's fifteen minutes. Thirty. We only want to do this test once. The doctor is precise and methodical, checking and double-checking. Right lung, left lung, back to the right, then left, just to be sure. It's half an hour with a nurse at my side — used to this role, I'm sure — holding my hand, steady, whispering "it's okay, relax, relax" whenever my muscles suddenly tighten. My throat convulsively constricts around the tube. I'm choking. Gagging.

"Shh," she says, wiping the involuntary tears from my cheeks. "Everything's going to be okay. Everything will be fine."

* * *

It's good news and it's bad news. Dr. Collins doesn't play the game with me, asking which one I'd rather have first. She just launches into the good: everything is clean. Sparkling. The single expensive, full-color, uncomfortable bronchoscopy has confirmed what multiple thrifty, black-and-white, simple X-rays were telling us all along. There are no infections in my lungs.

Dr. Collins smiles. She shrugs. She stands at the foot of my bed and does this little half smile, apologetic, because she knows that as good as the news is — *No infections! Woo-hoo!* — what it really means is that my Hickman is coming out. It has to. We're both reading between the lines. She's standing there, right, all cool and calm and collected, and it really is good news, that the myriad tests I've undergone recently have turned up nothing but nothing. But we both know where this is going.

Dr. Collins is standing at the foot of my bed and I'm trying to pretend like I don't have a fever. *Stupid. Stupid, Robert.* I'm shivering. Blankets are piled. She can read my charts. She knows better. I haven't been able to go, what, two consecutive days without spiking a temp above 105? I try, ineffectively, to keep my teeth from chattering while I wait for the Demerol to kick in. If it's not my lungs, then it's my clean, infection-free Hickman catheter. It's really not all that complicated. It's binary. A process of elimination. It *can't* be the Hickman, because it looks perfect; but then again, it can't *not* be, you know, because it's the only foreign object currently lodged in my body.

It's designed to be removed, with this clamp underneath my skin that somehow makes sure that there will be no additional bleeding when the long plastic tube is removed. A clamp that will stay with me, something you can feel under my skin on the upper part of my right chest, long after the Hickman is gone.

Dr. Collins doesn't need anesthesia. It's just a simple tug. I'd never pulled on the catheter hard enough (*never wanted to*), and she won't need to do much more than put one hand firmly on my chest, near the collarbone, another hand securely gripping the tube that extends out of my body.

One ... two ... three. *Yank*!

Done. Goodbye easy access to major arteries. This worries me a little, losing my Hickman. It's been, what, almost a month now since I've been neutropenic? Just about as long since I've been able to keep any food down. Even though it's great that we don't need my Hickman for any more chemo, my bone marrow still hasn't recovered yet. What happens if it never does? Wouldn't I need my catheter again in the near future if there was an emergency bone marrow transplant?

Probably. One day at a time, though. One problem at a time. This should help with the fevers, at least, which is the most important thing. It's immediately less convenient, no doubt: instead of being able to pop the needle into the free port at the end of my catheter for regular blood draws, we're back to slapping the inside of my arms. *Good veins, here.* Tight rubber around my upper arm, or my elbow. *Flex, please,* then relax as the needle finds a vein, somewhere, right arm, left arm, it doesn't really matter.

I don't care much about needles anymore. I'm finding it hard to care about much of anything anymore.

* * *

I'm having an equally hard time remembering things. Not the obvious stuff: my name, family members, today's date, the name of the current president, all that. It's not amnesia. I'm sleeping so much. I'm sleeping all the time, waking up, sleeping again. Sometimes I can't tell. Conversations are lost, stuff from yesterday, last week. Mornings and afternoons and evenings are repetitive. My days bleed together.

I don't know for sure if Dr. Collins ever explained that we'd need to be doing this test, but she probably did. She must have. It's about accuracy and precision, always, so I know she must have told me about this even if I can't remember when. We already know that I've got leukemia. We knew, before I'd left England, that it is a specific type: Acute Myeloid Leukemia. It is extremely aggressive.

Even the exact subtype has been clear through my various bone marrow biopsies. There are eight subtypes of AML, all with different symptoms and treatments, different methods of identification. Mine is the M3 subtype of AML. It's unique enough that Dr. Collins even calls it something slightly different: Acute Promyelocytic Leukemia, or APL. My earliest symptoms — especially the profuse bleeding — were fucking *textbook*.

And so, Dr. Collins patiently explains, we get to the purpose behind this latest test: based on everything we know to date it's obvious that I have the M3 subtype of AML. The confirmation of this, the official test that eliminates all possible doubt, is why we will now look to my DNA for answers.

I don't have any idea what she needed to extract to get the results of this latest test, or how complicated the process was to get to the desired results. Science is fucking awesome. That there's this much aggregate knowledge about leukemia is incredible. The word "cytogenetics" is used several times. I don't pretend to know much about genetics beyond some vague high school biology class recollections of Gregor Mendel and peas or pea pods or something, all the possible and impossible genetic combinations based on earlier generations. I don't even know what my DNA looks like. Links in a chain, I suppose. A double helix. It's all very comic-book like when I imagine the labs and the glowing vials and the swirling camera angles, mad scientists in crisp white coats and Thomas Dolby electric haircuts, cackling over what they've found in my DNA.

One of the things they're looking for — *one of the things they knew to look for* — they've found. Apparently there's a gene on my fifteenth chromosome, and another gene on my seventeenth chromosome that have swapped places.

"It's called translocation," Dr. Collins says.

It's a genetic mutation. She assures us that this mutation isn't hereditary, I probably wasn't even born with it, and if I ever have kids it won't pass down to them, either. But at some point over the past twenty years, for some unknown reason, two very specific genes on two very specific links in my genetic chain traded places. Turns out I'm a mutant, after all, although pretty much the opposite of Wolverine! You want to know why my body started to produce all sorts of wonky, immature, ineffective blood cells? Apparently, that was my mutant power a month or so ago.

Now we know. It doesn't change anything in terms of my treatment. Dr. Collins tells us that there are some new clinical trials based on some new research that show promising signs for treatment of APL patients. We're already past the point where we could have opted for one of those clinical trials, apparently, but it's good to know regardless.

For me, this new level of detail is another in a long line of similar diagnostic tests we've done. I'm happy for the accuracy. I'm glad my doctors are being thorough. For my mother, though, it is something else entirely. This DNA test makes my leukemia appear to be less than random. It is no longer a lightning bolt of bad news from the sky, an out-of-control city bus as I'm walking across the intersection. If this was in my DNA since birth, even if there's no conclusive research as to exactly how or why the translocation eventually takes place, then it's as if my own body has been waiting for two decades to spring this particular genetic trap.

* * *

Cindy will be gone for the weekend. It's mid-April, Easter Sunday coming up, and she's made plans to spend it with family in the small mountain town where she and her husband grew up. I'm surprised to see her early Saturday morning. She's waking me up, as usual, except she's not supposed to be here today. She's supposed to be on the road for her vacation. She's wearing shorts and a fleece jacket.

"I'm not here long," she says. "I have something I wanted to give you first." She hands me a bright yellow envelope. There are a couple of Snoopy and Woodstock stickers on the outside.

I sit up, as best as I can, to hug her.

"*Cindy*. Thank you. You didn't have to do this."

My two bulletin boards are completely filled with cards and notes and letters. I've shifted my Far Side calendar to the bottom, so that it's hanging over the edge, just to make room for more cards. The cards have come from all over — friends at Lancaster, immediately after I'd left, and, now that I've been in the hospital for nearly two months, follow-up cards to make sure everything is going well; friends from Carleton, sometimes sending a card a week; neighbors; former teachers; former classmates all the way back to elementary school; my parent's co-workers; daily cards from my Aunt.

I don't need (*or expect*) a get-well card from Cindy. She's with me almost every day. She's helped in countless ways. If I would have allowed myself time to think about it, I probably could have figured out that the reason my temps spiked the highest when she isn't working is because I've equated all of the good things that have happened since we'd arrived at the hospital — all of the healing that's been taking place — with her. *If Cindy isn't here*, my chemo-infused brain believes, *then I don't get better*.

"Careful," she says.

I've opened the envelope, carefully taking out the card.

"There's something inside," she says.

Already in the envelope I can see tiny metal dots, shiny punches of confetti. They're falling out of the card. A few fall into my hand before fluttering further downward, pinpoints of color on my white bed sheets. The outside of the card has Snoopy and Woodstock dancing together, hands held tightly, noses pointing skyward, their feet a circular blur. Inside, there are hundreds of bits of confetti. More fall out.

"Catch those," Cindy says. "Those are your blood counts!" She's written the same thing inside the card. We've been waiting almost a month, now, for my counts to return, for my bone marrow to do anything, and I wish it was simple as confetti inside an Easter card. It's the thought that counts. I know Cindy wants my counts to come back as badly as I do. I'll take them. I'll take absolutely anything at this point, even though these bits of colored paper won't show up on any of my charts.

"Thanks, Cindy. This means a lot to me."

"You're welcome. Now don't get another fever while I'm gone, okay?"

"No fevers this weekend, just for you," I say. We both know this is a lie.

She hugs me again. "Okay, then. I'll see you soon."

✳ ✳ ✳

Saturday and Sunday pass without incident. These things are the same. There is a sameness in my days, a kind of perpetual *déjà vu*, this magnetic pull from my bed that makes my limbs so heavy, my body not strong enough to want to bother with resistance. Let the heavy lids close. Let familiar sleep surround.

Drugs arrive in the morning. Benadryl to go along with the fresh pints of blood and platelets hanging next to my bed. Are Mom and

Paul here today or Dad and Jane? Laura? Scott? Blake? Who is with me today? Everybody? Nobody? I am sleepy. Sleepy sleep tempts me.

White coats are in and out of my room. They blur. The blurring blurs mumble to my parents, their voices in and out, a "Robert" here and a "patience" there, sentences sifting into my dreams, then jarring me awake, then coaxing me back down again. It's the same thing as yesterday. It's the same as last month.

I can feel the chills before they even start, like the driving line of a thunderstorm. A nurse who is not Cindy puts her fingers on my wrists, takes my temperature with great care, brings one steaming blanket, two, and even though she's doing everything right, nothing happens until the Demerol arrives a short while later. It's the same as it ever is: knees, chest, chattering chills, all followed by the rush of the push, the melting draining whoosh, and then I'm sleeping again until someone wakes me.

I drift sideways through the weekend, waiting for Cindy to return.

* * *

Rough hands are shaking me awake. Gentle hands, roughly. One of Cindy's slight but strong hands grabs my left wrist, the other pushes repeatedly against my left shoulder.

"Wake up, Robert! Wake up wake up wake up wake up wake up!"

She's back from the weekend and I'm happy to see her, but I'm so sleepy, too. There is no bright morning light trying to push through the curtains. The sun isn't even up yet. Cindy starts work early. Too early.

"Wake up, Robert," she says. "They're back!"

"I know you're back, Cindy. But it's so *early*."

"Not me," she laughs. "Your counts! Your polys are back."

It's just a blip. The tiniest of tiny blips on the chart, but there is a number, now, where for the past month there had been none. I'm all a million questions suddenly, wide awake, reaching for the controls at the side of my bed, fumbling for the little button that's like a triangle pointing up. I'd like to say that I'm sitting up in bed, like a bolt, but I'm still too tired for that. The bed adjusts. It's motorized, adjustable, and it helps me get kind of vertical without having to expend any energy.

"Are you sure?" I ask.

"Positive," Cindy says. "Absolutely positive."

"How many?"

"Twelve."

"That's it? That doesn't sound like much."

Cindy laughs. "It's better than zero."

"Are you sure?"

"Very sure."

"Could it be a mistake?"

"We'll do some extra blood draws today. We'll make sure."

It's so completely unexpected, this rough early morning wake-up call, these new counts coming back so late in the game. It's the best news we've had in a long time. It's probably the single best piece of news we've received since I've been in the hospital. But that still doesn't prevent me from asking the obvious question. Maybe I just want to hear Cindy say it out loud.

"This is good, right?"

"Yes, Robert," she says, smiling, laughing. "This is the best kind of good."

More counts return in the days that follow. Platelets are back. Polys creep higher. Hematocrit is up. Everything is up — except my temperatures, thankfully. As soon as my counts started to come back, the near-daily fevers stopped. It couldn't have been anything other than sudden, all this news, but it's still a surprise. It lightens everybody's mood. This is better news, by far, than knowing I'd achieved remission. If my counts are back, then that means my marrow is back, finally, once again producing healthy blood cells.

In a matter of days, the conversations have changed. We were all about a backup plan to our backup plan, discussions moving forward about an emergency bone marrow transplant — maybe even accepting a partial 4/6 match because it was the best we could find — because it had been looking more and more likely that my marrow would never recover on its own. Now, though, we're laying out the requirements for my departure. I'll still need to come back later in about a month, and then once more about a month after that for the rest of my protocol, two more rounds of consolidation chemotherapy, but I'll be allowed some time at home between those two rounds.

"Your counts will need to be at certain levels," Cindy tells me. "Dr. Collins will tell you more about it. There are a few minimum thresholds she'll want you to reach before you can go home. Not just the main counts, either. There'll be a lot of different factors she'll be looking at."

"How long?" I ask.

"Before you're back home?"

"Yeah. How long do you think it'll take before I can get out of here?"

"It depends," she says. "Depends on how quickly all of your counts recover. I wouldn't want to say. It'll be up to Dr. Collins."

"Can you guess?" I'm itching. I am so ready to get out of this hospital, back to my house, my bed, a neighborhood that I'm familiar with, a couple of different loops, a mile or two, that I can run or bike. Being able to get up and out of bed, to actually get dressed again, wearing something other than pajamas for once, to go out to restaurants, movies, whatever. Not to mention that it's less than two weeks until my twenty-first birthday. I can't wait.

Cindy smiles. "You're doing awesome, Robert. You really are. You'll be home soon enough."

"Next week?"

Now she laughs. "Just be patient. It won't be long, now."

* * *

Cindy is right, of course. The few remaining bumps before I'm out of the hospital are minor. With an across-the-board increase in my blood counts, the chemotherapy has pretty much worked its way out of my system. The fevers have vanished, which also means I'm not taking nearly as many meds throughout the day.

My appetite has finally returned, too. I'm surprised to find that I'm actually hungry again, that I'm thinking about getting some food into my system. Baby steps. I've been down this road before, tricked by drugs into believing that I'm ready to eat solid foods only to dash off to my bathroom. So I stick to the basics, steer towards the bland. The hospital continues to bring me three mostly square meals a day. I'll pick at the lightly toasted white bread, the saltine crackers, maybe nibbling at tiny cut up carrots or rubbery celery.

I'm trying to get more exercise during these days of rapid improvement, taking walks on my own through the deeper reaches of the hospital. Wheeling my little buddy into the middle of my cold floor, struggling to eke out a handful of sit-ups, or a single wobbly-armed push-up. I'll visit the cafeteria once a day or so, rooting through the vending machines. Potato chips, Kit Kats, even the occasional can of Coke. It's all good. I can actually taste it, and everything stays down.

Every day, now, I'm feeling better than the last. No hesitation, no qualifications. Everybody is in a good mood as we watch my counts tick higher and higher. Last week seems like forever ago, even though I can see it clearly marked on my calendar. I'd stopped blacking out the numbers when we started my second week of chemo — I think I wanted to know for sure what the days were, how many days had transpired. Since then, I've circled the days after they passed.

Throughout March I'd also written out some shorthand on the left-hand side, down the column of Sundays, a reminder of how long it had been. "DAY 1" was on my first Monday of chemo, March 5th. "DAY 7" is on the Sunday after that, with "DAY 14" and "DAY 21" closing out the month. Into April I'd changed it up again, using a small blue felt-tip to continue the pattern: 28 on the first, then 35, then 42 on Easter Sunday. 49 days now. Seven weeks since I'd arrived on a flight from London. When you add the ten days I'd spent in hospitals in Lancaster and London before that, it's been two full months since I've slept anywhere other than a hospital bed. I am itching to get out.

When Dr. Collins comes into my room, later, I'm happy that we're finally beyond talking about what we need to do to get through today. We're starting to sketch out some long-term goals. Some future timelines, weeks and months away. She pulls my calendar down from the corkboard for reference. She lays it out along the foot of my bed. I bring my knees up so I can still see; Mom slides her chair closer for a better view.

"We're expecting you'll be able to leave sometime around here" Dr. Collins says, using two fingers as a kind of pointer, a couple of big swirls covering the last weeks of April. "You'll go home for much-needed rest. We'll miss you, and we might want you to come back once or twice, primarily for blood work, just to keep an eye on things, understand."

I am so excited. Nervous, excited, pent-up energy makes my feet twitch so much that the bed is shaking. Mom reaches her hand over and pushes gently down on my knees.

"Please," she says.

"Sorry," I say, trying to settle my legs down.

Dr. Collins continues. "Assuming your counts keep moving the way we think they will, Robert, you should be home by the end of the month. Let's plan on a couple two, maybe three weeks at home to rest and recover." She flips the calendar ahead to May. She looks to Mom, then back to me, then to the calendar again. "Here," she says, tapping on the fourteenth. Monday. Smack dab in the middle of the month.

"We're going to need to plan ahead, to schedule a few things before you come back. But this looks like a good day to start your second round, Robert. Your first consolidation round. Now that we have the leukemia on the run, we're going to give you a few more weeks to build up your strength before we hit it again."

I look closer at the unblemished calendar. May 14th. I notice that it's the day after Mother's Day. I'm sure Mom has already seen that, too. Even still, I can't wait to get home. It's hard to fathom that I'm almost there!

CHAPTER 24

The house where I grew up is simple and unremarkable. It's wedged in between many other houses of similar shapes and sizes, stretching out for several miles not too far from the high school. Lots of chain link fences. Some well-maintained lawns, but lots of brown, weedy patches.

There used to be woods a few blocks away, years ago, at the end of a kind of cul-de-sac, just up the hill. I'd take my bike through those woods for a fun shortcut to the grocery store. They also proved to be great cover back in grade school when Ian and I would throw on several layers of clothing and — because we weren't *idiots* — protective goggles for our summer BB gun wars. The woods are long gone, now, paved over to make room for more roads and parks and houses.

Our house is in the middle of the block, on the south side of the street. The road is straight, here, but it curves off sharply to the right as you head downhill. The lawn is small and tidy. A sort of rock garden cuts an arc halfway through the yard. Mom has planted a number of plants and flowers on the top part of the yard, including rose bushes. There's a young maple tree near the edge of the front sidewalk, close to the street, and a long, low evergreen-type of a shrub that follows along the sidewalk to the house. This helps to create some natural separation between the driveway — leading down to a small, single-car tuck-under garage — and the rest of the yard. We used to have grass on the far side of the driveway, too, a thin strip of difficult-to-maintain lawn that was eventually paved over.

This is such a beautiful, welcome sight.

I have never been away from home for this long. And I can't quite describe how wonderful it feels standing just inside the doorway, since I've technically been back "home" for almost two months now. It doesn't count unless you walk through the front door. Being home doesn't count unless you're really home.

The air is a little damp, but surprisingly nice for late April. It smells amazing. I'm standing here inhaling the familiar smells of home, so completely thrilled that it's nothing like the room I'd left this morning that I begin to laugh. Even better is the fact that nobody will interrupt my sleep at all hours of the night to swallow a pill, or check my pulse, or quietly try to change out a bag of antibiotics while not waking me up. I won't need to leave any lights on. Sleeping through the night, in complete darkness? I'm ecstatic.

But first: I've got to tackle the stairs leading to the main landing. This shouldn't be so intimidating. My bony arms are poking out from underneath the Pendle College tee-shirt Simon had given me before I'd left Lancaster. My legs are even more twig-like. It feels like they aren't much bigger than my arms at this point, so weak, so emaciated.

There aren't many stairs in front of me. It's a split-level landing, one set of stairs, maybe eight or ten, heading up to the main floor. That's basically the one level for all the rooms in the house: living room, kitchen, dining room, three bedrooms and a shared bathroom. The other set of stairs, lined with a wooden rail, leads to the garage and unfinished basement. Years ago, Mom had to get creative about making ends meet. That meant ordering a cord of wood to augment winter heating— or maybe just half a cord, depending on how much we'd had left over from the previous year. We'd see if we could go all winter without ever turning on the heat. The wood was stacked outside, along the west side of the house, protected from generally mild Seattle winters by a thick green tarp.

Once a week, at least, I'd push a full wheelbarrow through the garage, down through the narrow basement hallway, creating a second, smaller stack in the southeast corner of the house. I'd dump the wood on the cool concrete. This was my work area. I'd first break apart the larger pieces with a maul, tapping it down into the soft wood before swinging both the wood and maul together in one wide sweep. The wood broke apart on the hard concrete floor of the basement. I'd use a smaller hand ax from there for kindling. Besides being a practical way to get the firewood we needed to heat the house, it was also a great workout. I loved it. My hands would blister and callous. My battered, paint-spattered boombox would be plugged into one of the outlets next to the window that looked out into our back yard.

Even then, my arms weren't exactly huge, but chopping firewood made them strong. My legs, too, from all the wheeling and lifting and squatting and bracing for the wide swing of the maul. Biking for miles from the house to the grocery store, or to school, or even all the way down the hill to Southcenter. It wasn't so long ago when I would bound upstairs from the basement two or three steps at a time. There's no way my legs are ready for that now. Let's just try making it up one, shall we?

Mom looks down from the top of the landing. Paul has come to my level, offering a helping hand.

"You doing okay?" he asks. "Need some help?"

I laugh again. It seems so ridiculous that I'm worried I can't even make it up this one flight of stairs without stopping to catch my breath. I'm home again. That's all that matters. "I'm good," I say, and I mean it.

It's so good to be home. These first few days take time, though. They are a difficult adjustment. My legs are noticeably sore, still, just walking up and down the stairs, so fucking exhausted from the rudimentary act of walking outside to check the mail. It takes a few days for me to get used to even simple movement from my bedroom to the kitchen to the couch and back.

I'm inspired to try a short run around the neighborhood. This is a mistake. I can barely get to the end of the block. It's only been two months since I'd left Lancaster and my legs are weak and withered. A short loop outside of my bedroom window at Lancaster seems like a luxury, now, a level of fitness I wish I had back.

I tell myself, initially, to just take it easy. I don't need to push too hard, too soon. It's enough to sleep in my own bed. To wake up when I want to, shuffle to the kitchen with a blanket wrapped around my shoulders because I'm still so cold most of the time and pour a bowl of cereal for breakfast. *My own bowl. My* decision about when and what to do for breakfast. I'll carry that bowl to the living room and set it on the coffee table if I want, watching senseless morning television. There are no doctors or nurses constantly coming into my room to take my temperature or check on how I'm doing. I'll finish my cereal and stretch out on the couch and maybe take a mid-morning nap before trying to figure out what to do with the rest of my day.

We're already focusing so much on my weight loss that it's not enough to have a bowl of cereal for breakfast. I'm down to 145 pounds. That's twenty pounds gone, and it shows. We all know how important it is for me to regain as much of that as I can when I'm at home, so with every meal I also have a tall glass of Carnation Instant Breakfast. It's like chocolate milk, only with an abundance of additional calories. I need all the calories I can get these days.

These are easy days: rest, eat, sleep, repeat.

Everything has been so precise, so regimented, so scheduled for the past two months that I hardly know what to do. To help pass the time, I decide to sift through the large cardboard box that was in the middle of my bedroom when I'd come home a few days ago. It was addressed to me, in handwriting that I didn't recognize, postmarked from Lancaster, England. It was sent a good month ago. I'd tried to jog my memory when I first saw it. Had Mom mentioned it before? She was always so great about bringing any cards or letters that had been accidentally sent to the house, I can't imagine she would have forgotten to bring this on one of her visits to the UWMC.

It wasn't until I'd taken a pair of scissors from my desk and cut through the packing tape to peer inside the box that I remembered what this was. We'd left in such a hurry. I'd had to leave so many things behind, and now they've been returned. Simon must have packed all of this for me. A few textbooks, plus copies of *Pride and Prejudice*, *Jude the Obscure*, and *Bleak House*. Clothes and tapes that were left behind in the rush to get me back home. It feels like forever ago. Wayne might have helped pack it, too. School notebooks. Loose papers. Photographs from my bookshelf: stacks of photos from trips to the Lake District, to York, stupid smiling late nights at the JCR with the boys. A clean and folded Pendle college tee-shirt. Pens, coffee cups, loose change that I'll never have a chance to spend in this country.

What am I to do with all of this? It's important, but it's from a life that's already forever out of my reach. I've closed that chapter. Abruptly. Permanently. I'm not at Lancaster and I'm not at Carleton and I'm certainly not at the University of Washington Medical Center, the place, most recently, that has given me clear purpose and razor-sharp focus. I'm in between everything.

That's what's so hard about these first days. It's not just the lingering fatigue and lack of stamina, which of course I should have expected. It's so cold and damp, too. No matter how many layers I wear I can't seem to get warm. I'll pick around the edges of my meals, waiting patiently for my appetite to return in full along with my energy and strength, drinking extra calories from a tall glass in the meantime.

I've been desperate to come home and now that I'm finally here I have no idea what to do with myself.

* * *

Ian calls the house. He just happens to be in Seattle for a few days before returning to Reed for spring term. On a lark, he thought he'd give me a call to see if I was available to get together.

Wasn't sure what the spring break schedule was like for Carleton, or if I was even back yet from England, but thought it was worth a roll of the dice to call.

"It's really good to hear your voice," he says. "How have you been? What have you been up to?"

It's been at least a year since we've last seen one another. Maybe closer to two and a half, another one of his brief trips back from Alaska. That visit had involved a weekend in Vancouver, British Columbia — around New Year's, during winter break of my freshman year at Carleton. We took turns attempting to break land speed records in his Saab Turbo on the drive back to Seattle.

She likes to run free, Ian had said, smiling. *Somewhere between 90 and 95 miles per hour is when she really purrs.* I've never driven as fast for as far as Ian and I did on that trip.

Since then, though, there'd been maybe the occasional letter or phone call. It's tough to stay in touch when we go to colleges in Oregon and Minnesota, and return trips home are to Alaska, and Washington, respectively, but we've tried.

"Did you have a good spring break? How was Lancaster?"

I'm still not very good at this. Wasn't good at it in Lancaster. Didn't get any better with more practice at the University of Washington Medical Center. How do you shift from mundane banter with friends to conversations about cancer?

And Ian is a *great* friend. Probably one of my best ever. Even though we've known each other most of our lives, we've only been able to stay in casual contact since his family moved back to Alaska. We've been friends since, what, fourth grade? Maybe fifth? Ian is a year younger than me and we'd bounced around between a few different elementary schools in Renton as the Gifted Child

Program struggled to find a permanent home. There were early mornings together playing *Asteroids* on the cutting-edge Atari 2600 at his house before school. Afternoons and weekends trying other games: *Dungeons and Dragons*, *Anti-Monopoly*, *Ace of Aces*, or even blackjack and poker in a makeshift casino we'd built in his backyard. We'd spent a few fantastic summers together at Camp Orkila on Orcas Island, too. Ian has been my oldest, most constant friend, regardless of whether or not we're living in the same state.

I'm thrilled that he's called. But how do I answer his questions? *What have I been up to? How was my spring break?* I guess it just needs to be the truth.

"No spring break this year," I say. "I just got out the hospital. I mean, like only a handful of days ago. Lancaster was great except for when I found out I had leukemia. Now I'm home for a few weeks before I have to go back to the hospital for another round of chemo."

"What?" Ian asks. "You what? What?"

I doubt that these conversations will get any easier as the spring and summer progresses. It's a flood of explanations to Ian, feeble attempts at humor, at defusing an already tense conversation. I don't know how to talk about my leukemia. I want to gloss over the shitty times from earlier in the month and focus on the fact that I'm in remission. I'm cancer-free. I spend so much time fretting about how Ian is reacting to this news that I lose sight of the fact that he's extraordinarily worried about me.

We make plans to meet up tomorrow.

"Are you okay to go out?" he asks. "We can head to Southcenter or something. Maybe grab some lunch? Or catch a movie? Is that okay? Is that safe?"

I tell him that would be outstanding. Amazingly outstanding. It'd be great to get outside some more, even if it is just down the hill to the mall. It will be a welcome change.

✳ ✳ ✳

My counts haven't returned completely, and my legs are still scrawny toothpicks, but it feels so good to be getting out of the house. The drive down the valley is great. Knowing that I'll have a chance to visit with an old friend is great. The cold and damp of a spring afternoon in Seattle isn't great, but I'm not sure if that isn't just me. It's so hard to keep warm these past days. I crank the heat in my truck on my way to Southcenter.

We're planning to meet at the recently renovated food court before the movie. If we even get to the movie. But I need to find a bathroom, first. You'd think there'd be one nearby. I'm either stupid or blind or both, and I end up meandering farther away from the food court than I'd expected.

I've got to admit that I don't have much swagger. I'm not so much angry, not anymore, as I'm just fucking tired. But I'm trying to be observant, trying to pay attention to my surroundings. The bathrooms must be somewhere. This is practically my back yard growing up, this mall, and it's entirely possible that I might bump into somebody else from high school, or even grade school, and find myself trying to explain my appearance.

I haven't yet learned to lie about the hairless head, the scrawny pipes poking out from underneath whatever loose and ill-fitting tee-shirt I'd thrown on that morning, the equally baggy, ratty jeans with a belt notched as tight as possible and still barely keeping those jeans on my hips. I dread the questions, the pitying looks, the awkward silence that stretches interminably as old acquaintances try to figure out polite ways to end the conversation and move on.

"What?" I ask.

Two girls have just walked past me. One is brunette, the other blond, well-dressed, each holding bags from Nordstrom's and The Gap. They're about my age. They might even be former classmates. Maybe friends of friends who know me by reputation. They'd said something to me as they passed by. I couldn't really tell, because I'm too busy being observant but they definitely said something. They ignore me at first, so I turn and follow them for a few steps to make sure they'd heard my question.

"I'm sorry. Did you say something?"

They might be cute. I'm thinking that they might possibly be cute, and maybe former classmates or something, and I don't really have to get into a detailed explanation about the hair and the skinny arms or anything. They could just get all doe-eyed and say *wow, Robert, it's been awhile but you look great, really great*, and I'll be all *shucks, gosh, thanks* and then I'd invite them back to the food court where Ian and I can sit with them and catch up on old times together in the warm light of the afternoon sun.

They turn on their tip-toes. It's weird. Kind of an outside in thing, timed perfectly, both pivoting at the same time, almost brushing shoulders as they stop and look back at me. Like something they've practiced. Like something they've totally done, like, a million times before.

The brunette speaks up. Her face is icy scorn.

"You heard me," she says.

"No, really. I ..."

"You people make me fucking sick," she says. "Why don't you go fuck yourself?"

They turn again — toes, timing, everything — and casually walk away. Heads together, giggling, laughing. One last look back at me, the blond this time, flipping me off with her free hand, slowly mouthing two words. She enunciates her silence, making sure that I'm able to read her lips: *fuh-king skin head.*

CHAPTER 25

A couple of days later and I'm meeting up with Scott and Blake at the TGI Friday's in Kirkland to celebrate my twenty-first birthday. Ian had to head back to college already, otherwise he'd be here, too, continuing our conversation (*and stunned disbelief*) that in addition to all the other shit I've been dealing with now we need to add being mistaken for a racist neo-Nazi to the pile. Guess I need to start wearing more popped collar polo shirts and Madras shorts when I go to the mall instead of white tee-shirts and jeans.

Scott and Blake and I will have a beer or two here before heading out for the rest of the night. I'm not sure what we're going to do. Maybe walk down to the Kirkland waterfront and check out a few new bars that Blake has heard good things about. Or we'll drive across the bridge to downtown Seattle, parking somewhere near Pioneer Square to explore several options there.

I don't really care where we go or what we do. How late we stay out. I'm just ecstatic about the contrast. I'd spent far too much time in front of the mirror earlier, trying to figure out what to wear, striving for that delicate balance between casual indifference and still being so fucking self-conscious about my weight and hair —

or lack thereof, in both departments. I *feel* healthy, though. I feel stronger than I have in months.

There was no arguing with my mirror, though: I look like shit. I'm maybe a buck fifty, soaking wet. And what to do about my head? Do I wear a baseball cap or not? Do I hide the obvious baldness? Or should I just embrace it, confident in the knowledge that this is who I am, that this is part of my story, and that it really doesn't matter what other people think anyway? In the end, I'd settled for as preppy as I can from what's in my closet: a kind of light purple polo shirt, untucked, hanging loosely over a pair of khaki shorts. I shouldn't care what other people think but I do. I don't want this night to be ruined by somebody else's ignorance. I'm not wearing anything on my head. I figure it's just going to be mostly my buddies and I anyway, hopefully. I'm not expecting to have to interact with anybody.

It's not quite 5:00 yet. Were we meeting at five or six? I don't remember. I order a pint of Guinness at the bar — a conscious nod toward my friends at Lancaster, ordering my Pendle College "usual" — and leaf through the menu checking out appetizers. I'm not hungry, but I know I need to eat. Every calorie matters. I get the bartender's attention and ask if he can throw some chicken wings onto my order.

The bar is slowly filling up with a young, well dressed crowd. A guy who doesn't look much more than a handful of years older than me smokes a cigarette off to my left. He's wearing a dark suit, tie loosened at the collar. Short, slicked hair. He was there when I'd first arrived, sitting alone, drinking a mixed drink from a tall glass. Bourbon and coke, maybe? He's glanced in my direction a few times but I mostly ignore him.

He puts out his cigarette and gets up as if he's leaving but grabs his half-full glass instead and comes around the corner of the bar to sit next to me.

"Hey," he says. It's obvious, after just one word, that this isn't his first drink of the afternoon. "I got a question: why'd you do that to your head?"

This is the first time a stranger has taken the time to ask me about how I look. I don't know quite how to react, have even less of an idea what to say. *This is why I should have worn the baseball cap.* So much simpler to just sit quietly and anonymously and drink my beer while waiting for Scott and Blake to show up. But now I have to say something. The truth, still, is easiest.

"I have leukemia," I tell him. "It's kind of like cancer."

"Really?" he says. "No fucking shit. Really?"

I tell him that it's true, then give a few cursory details. Diagnosed a couple of months ago, lots of time in the hospital, lots of shitty chemo, even worse complications. Just got out last week. But I'm fine now, it's all good, in remission, prognosis awesome for full recovery. It's my birthday. Twenty-one. Just out to celebrate with a quiet night with my buddies.

He doesn't take his eyes off me while I share all of this. Finishing off his drink, he waves the bartender over. "What are you having, man? Guinness? I'm buying."

I protest, but he's insistent. What follows is a barrage of semi-random questions: will my hair grow back, if it does will it be the same color, is cancer contagious, did I think I was going to die, did I throw up a lot, can I still, you know, have sex?

"Man," he sighs. There is silence after my answers, and he looks down at the bar.

Before I have a chance to excuse myself to get up and look for Scott and Blake, he launches into his life story. Or at least the most recent, most traumatic event: his fiancée had left him at the altar during the previous summer. Childhood sweethearts, they'd pictured spending the rest of their lives together from nearly the moment they'd met. They'd planned this huge wedding together a few years after they both finished college, an enormous crowd of people – mostly to please her parents, from the sounds of it. That meant hundreds of wedding guests murmuring at the church, watching him stand awkwardly, shifting from foot to foot while his one true love never walked down the aisle.

"Can you imagine the embarrassment, man? And the hurt? Fuck! It still pisses me off. She's talked with me a bit since. I mean, she apologized and everything, but we really haven't spoken at all after that day. I can't stomach seeing her."

"I can't imagine," I say.

He looks like he wants to cry, but he's smiling, too.

"You can't imagine?" he says. "I can't even *begin* to imagine what it's like to be in your shoes. I mean, I thought my life was fucked up. I thought I had it bad. Thanks, man. Seriously. You've shown me that as bad as that day was, it could have been so much worse."

We both take a slow drink of our beverages. We are both lost in thought.

"Fuck me," he says after a moment, more to his empty glass than to me. "I could have had cancer."

CHAPTER 26

Mom drives me back up to the hospital. We've been counting down to this day — I have it circled on my calendar, and I know she can't shake this bad feeling about the whole process. I can't believe how fast these past weeks have flown by.

"Look at you," she says as we pack up the trunk of her Mitsubishi with all sorts of stuff I think I might need over the course of the next month: books and my Nintendo and a half-dozen tapes for my Walkman and some blank journals, just in case. I might want to write something down. My birthday present from Dad and Jane, too, a white Toshiba laptop. Much better for writing. I want to be prepared.

I've decided to be more alert and active this time, too, so I've thrown some gym shorts and tee shirts and running shoes into my suitcase to go along with the always-comfortable pajamas. I'm even bringing along a couple of 20-pound dumbbells. I figure I can replicate my simple living room lifting routine in the corner of my new hospital room. I've got lots of upper body work to do, assuming I won't be sleeping or puking or fighting fevers.

"I mean, just look at you," Mom says, fighting back tears. "I know we need to go back, but you're just finally looking healthy again. It just doesn't make sense."

"What doesn't?"

"You look better than you have in months. So much better than when I came to get you in Lancaster. You're healthy, Robert, and strong. And now I'm taking you back to the hospital so Dr. Collins can make you sick again."

I don't argue the point. Of course that's not what my second round of chemo is for, and we both know it. I'm in remission but I'm not cured. Dr. Collins had explained all of this to us, several times, that after this round of chemo there'd still need to be at least one more.

But Mom's right, too. I've spent the better part of my time at home doing everything I can to get as strong as possible for this next month. I expect that this chemo is going to kick the shit out of me again. I just want to be ready for it. I want to be in and out in four weeks. I want my body to do a better job of sticking to the plans that Dr. Collins has laid out for it. The disconnect for Mom is that this isn't how hospitals are supposed to work. You don't drive your (*mostly*) perfectly healthy child to the hospital so that the talented doctors and nurses can give him a steady diet of toxic chemicals in order to knock out his immune system. We both need to remember that I am *not* cured yet, though. These are the steps we need to take to get there.

It's a quiet drive north along 405. We make it quickly through Bellevue before turning west onto 520. The highway bends and loops, down into a small valley south of Kirkland, and then a gradual twisting uphill to take us to the edge of Lake Washington.

It's a bright, sun-drenched day. As we come down onto the floating bridge deck, everything is unbelievable gorgeous: the broad expanse of lake on either side of the highway — short, choppy waves to the north, smooth as glass to the south. Looks like boaters are out in force, enjoying the fantastic spring morning. The Olympics stand tall, well in the distance beyond the low hills in front of us.

Days like today? These are the days where Seattle reminds you of the spectacular, almost commonplace beauty of living here.

The highway runs straight across the lake before picking up again, slightly, curving toward the U. It's easy to make out Husky Stadium getting closer, jutting up against the far west edge of the lake. And, because I'm looking for it — because I know, now, that it exists — the dim outline of the University of Washington Medical Center hiding behind the stadium. *Almost there.*

Mom's hands have been tight on the steering wheel. She looks over at me when we exit onto Montlake. We're close now, tires vibrating on the drawbridge grate, only a few stoplights away from the underground parking lot that connects to my hospital, an elevator to the sixth floor, and to Cindy and Anne and everything else. We make our way across the Montlake Cut.

I'm surprised when Mom reaches across the front seat to hold my left hand. Her hand is sweaty. Mine is too, maybe. Maybe probably.

"Well," I say. "We're back."

CHAPTER 27

My room is on the opposite side of the hospital. Instead of taking a sharp left turn down the hallway as we'd approached the main desk, coming in from the elevators, Mom and I are guided straight ahead. It's still a left turn at the end of that hallway, then, and only a couple of doors down. Now my view faces to the west, with no chance to see the Olympics beyond the many hills surrounding the University of Washington. Boats cruise up and down the Montlake Cut, making their way between the fresh water of Lake Washington and the salt water of Elliot Bay.

There's so much less activity this time. It's just Mom and I, ready to meet with Dr. Collins and her usual crowd of earnest med students when they come through for morning rounds. There's no hustle or bustle, no flurry of activity, no stress or worry.

I'm happy to see Dr. Collins again. It's good to be back.

"First of all," Dr. Collins tells me, "before you get too comfortable, you're going to visit Dr. Hickman again, later this morning. We're going to need that catheter again before we can start your consolidation round of chemotherapy."

I'd almost forgotten about needing another Hickman catheter. I mean, I'd *wanted* to forget about it. I'd wanted to push the memory of that unbelievably painful procedure (and the bleeding that followed) far, far away. That's not realistic, though. I know how vital it was for most of my treatment the past couple of months, and the same reasons I'd need to get one when I first arrived from England exist today. I've got another week of chemotherapy ahead of me. And more later in the summer. There's no way I could do that without a new catheter. I hadn't forgotten about it at all, but I haven't exactly been looking forward to it, either.

"And what about his chemo this time?" Mom asks. "Is it the same as before?"

"Identical," Dr. Collins says. "Seven and three. The exact same dosage and duration that we'd started you off with, Robert. We'll start after you get your new Hickman."

This all seems so simple, so mundane. We're getting ready to pump ara-C and daunorubicin into my body again, twenty-four hours a day, for a full seven days, and I'm actually feeling anxious to get started. Not for fear of the side-effects, which I'm well aware of, or that the chemo won't work like it did the first time. I'm anxious to get started so I don't lose any more days of a potentially beautiful Seattle summer all cooped up inside the hospital.

* * *

My schedule is completely different now. It's upside-down. Backwards. It's not the chemo. That's been surprisingly easy this time. All of the chaos that had surrounded me when I'd first arrived is gone now. I don't exactly like using the words "easy" and "chemo" together, but that's what it's been like so far. I know what to expect.

Even getting my replacement Hickman — it hurt like hell again, of course, but there's no internal bleeding after this one. Much of that is thanks to the fact that I'm in remission, now, have been since March, and am infinitely better off than I was at the beginning of all this. That things seem comparatively easy now is one of the benefits of starting a week of chemotherapy when your body is actually producing healthy blood cells.

This hospital is a familiar and comfortable place, precisely where I need to be to beat this thing. My schedule is all turned around because Cindy is working the night shift. It's a mandatory thing, apparently, something she needs to do for one month out of the year. There's a rotation that's set up. All of the nurses on the floor end up working overnights at least once. Things are generally quieter overnight, but not always.

We'd established a pattern during my first round in the hospital, right, where I'd wake up in the morning and Cindy would be there. The rest of the morning might be a fog of sleep and fevers and blood draws, but I'd trust that she was there to give me my meds. As the day progressed, and Anne's shift started, Cindy would hand off the baton. More often than not, I'd be asleep well before the transition from Anne's shift to the third shift. What can I do? It's not up to me to set the scheduling. Now it's Anne in the afternoon and evening, handing me off to Cindy for overnights. I want to be *awake* when Cindy is here.

The chemo is easy. I've got that licked. But this schedule change is throwing me for a loop. I'm none too happy about it. The solution ends up being pretty simple: I just stay up late. It's not like I have to get up in the morning for work or school. What's to keep me from shifting my schedule a bit, too? There's always plenty of lousy late-night TV worth watching, or overdue final essays from Lancaster that need to be written, so I can pass the time before she comes back to check my temps or mark more numbers on my chart.

Over the few weeks at home I'd gotten into something of a habit of exercising in front of the TV. Nothing major. It just felt too lazy to be sitting on the couch watching television for a couple of hours during the day. I was also frankly too exhausted, especially during that first week, to be able to do anything significant. So I'd just work in some push-ups and sit-ups during the commercials. There would be these short three to five-minute bursts. Eventually I'd bring in some light weights, some dumbbells, and get through a hybrid homemade workout to build back the strength I'd lost. I'll do that, too, as a way to keep active and awake during Cindy's shift.

Letterman would have been over for hours, and I'm just flipping up through the cable channels. My eyes are heavy. There'll be a movie, somewhere, that I can settle on before easing myself out of bed. I'm sure I'll fall asleep if I don't get up. The movie is background noise and it's late. Instead, I reach out for my "little buddy," always close by. Bags of chemo are hung carefully, long, clear tubes snaking their way into my chest. Push-ups are a little tricky. Not too bad, but tricky, still, when I'm that much more conscious of my catheter, and the length of tubing extending out from underneath my tee-shirt. Sit-ups are easier.

After the movie ends, I'll take a break and walk down the quiet halls, maybe one or two laps around the floor. It doesn't take too long before I'm resting and exercising and watching movies until dawn.

I'll sleep until noon or so, very much your stereotypical college kid home for break. This allows me to be alert and awake for when Anne's shift starts later in the day, and also works well for timing when my visitors usually drop by. They don't come as frequently as before. Everything about this consolidation round has been surprisingly easy. *Knock on wood.*

✳ ✳ ✳

Weeks later and I'm continuing to feel great. I've only had one fever that I can remember, and that wasn't all that high. Vomiting from the chemo was short lived, mostly near the end of that first week. Am I tired? Hell, yes. Fatigue is ever-present, and not just because I've been staying up so late. All things considered, though, it's been a walk in the park. It's been textbook: feeling kind of okay throughout my waking hours, with familiar side-effects that are mild at best. I haven't lost nearly as much weight as last time, either. I've been making a conscious effort to keep exercising every day.

One of my sophomore year roommates, Adam, had taught me this great method when I'd visited him in London earlier in the year. A fellow English major, he'd started his own Carleton study abroad program the January after I'd been at Lancaster. I'd crashed with him for a couple of nights after making my way back up from Greece during winter break.

Adam was an inspiration when it came to working out. He could find a way to get exercise in, no matter how small or cramped his dorm room in London. He showed me this one morning before we started a day of visiting tourist destinations like Trafalgar Square, the National Portrait Gallery, Big Ben, and Westminster Abbey.

You get a deck of cards. This helps break up the monotony of push-ups and sit-ups: shuffle a deck of cards and flip a card over. That's how many push-ups you do. Flip another card and that's your count for sit-ups. Keep flipping until you burn through the deck. Face cards count for ten. Aces, if you want to push yourself, are twenty. If you really want to push it, which Adam always does, then a deuce isn't a nice break where you only have to do two. It means you *double* the next card and do that number of push-ups or sit-ups instead.

It helps to make something of a game of these simple, effective body-weight exercises. And since I don't really know what the weeks after my chemo will be like, I work my way through a deck of cards every day. I'm standing in front of the window, swinging dumbbells up and down. Left arm, right arm. I'm careful, okay, making sure not to get the weights caught up with the clear tube snaking out of my chest. It feels impossible for me to get enough exercise during this month. I'm working against my cancer.

My walks through the hallway have more purpose than before. I'm not just shuffling along, trying to keep my legs from degenerating into barely functioning sticks of lean muscle. This time I get out of my room for real exercise, up and down the halls.

There's an exercise bike at the far end of my hallway. You make your way past the last set of rooms, and before the path dead-ends at the end of the building, there's a nice stretch of double windows. A bicycle is there for the patients to use. You could rotate the bike, I suppose, to face one window or the other. I like to aim it down the opposite hallway, though, windows on either side, staring down an imaginary track. My little buddy is next to me. If I pedal too fast, the tubes underneath my shirt — snaking down and out from my Hickman catheter — bounce lightly up and down on my thighs. As much as I'm *feeling* great, the reality is that neither my legs nor my lungs are up to speed yet.

I jack up the volume on my Walkman, dial down the resistance on the bike so it's not too impossibly difficult, and get to work. I'm imagining what it will be like to be doing this outside again. My quads and calves burn. Sweat drips from my forehead onto a white hospital towel I've spread out over the handlebars. My breathing is ragged and labored. I need to keep pushing myself.

As long as I'm physically capable of this kind of exertion, I'm going to do everything I can to get as strong as I can for whatever the rest of the summer has in store for me.

* * *

I've made a new friend, surprisingly, here on the floor. I'd been reluctant to socialize much for kind of the same reasons as before. Each of us tends to live in isolation to a certain degree. That's by necessity. Any number of us on this floor might have compromised immune systems. Or we're dealing with our own mortality in our own ways. And as much as I welcome and appreciate all of the visitors that come to my room on a regular basis, I haven't exactly tried to get to know any of the people around me. It's come as a pleasant surprise that I've become friends with my next door neighbor.

The other day I'd thrown on some shorts and a tee-shirt, a backwards Mariners ballcap to help minimize sweating into my eyes, a towel from my bathroom, my ever-present Walkman. I was pulling my little buddy out the door to get more time in on the exercise bike when I almost bumped into my neighbor crossing paths in the hallway. He looked about my age, maybe late twenties instead of early twenties. His hair was cut short but hadn't started to fall out yet. He, too, was pushing a small rolling cart loaded with familiar-looking bags of antibiotics and chemo. He wore a faded Mariners tee-shirt over a pair of black sweats.

"Nice shirt," I'd said. "Excellent taste!"

"Yes! You, too. Is that your room?"

"It is. I'm Robert."

"Eric."

I started to reach to shake his hand but remembered. I rubbed my bald head instead. "I'm in for leukemia—AML. My second round of chemo. You?"

"Leukemia, too. ALL. This is all very new to me."

"You heading out for a walk? Interested in some company?"

"Wasn't planning to, but sure. Just a sec." He'd taken a step back into his room and called out to a young woman I hadn't noticed before. She was sitting on the edge of his bed. "Jen? Hon? I'm just going to go out for a bit. I'll be back soon."

We only walked for a couple of laps that first time. I'd guessed right: he's twenty-seven years old, which is unusual for ALL. Acute Lymphoblastic Leukemia is far more common in children. He explained that typical chemo for a patient with ALL is much lower dosage than what he's getting, usually paced out once or twice a week, often lasting for years. His treatment was different. It would require a bone marrow transplant. Fortunately, his younger brother was a perfect match. His chemo — much like mine — was meant to immediately induce remission. Once in remission, he'd begin the bone marrow transfer process, probably transferring to Fred Hutchinson for that.

He and his wife, Jen, live on the other side of the mountains in Spokane. She's staying at a Best Western near the University but spends most of her days and nights with Eric. I don't ask if they have any kids. It doesn't sound like it. "It's tough," he tells me, "being all the way out here. Don't get me wrong. The company is great. It's just that it's too far for most of our friends and family to visit. It's easily a four or five hour drive from Spokane, depending on traffic. My mom and dad have been coming out every weekend. The rest of the time, though, it's usually just Jen and me. And I'm already getting a little stir crazy!"

It's easy to empathize with Eric. He gets it. More so than any of my friends or family who have been incredibly supportive, Eric understands what it's like. And with that we start visiting each other regularly.

Sometimes we'll walk. We don't leave the floor, of course, but it's still good to get out of our rooms. I'll invite him over to watch movies together. I introduce him to Scott and Blake when they visit in the afternoon. We'll fire up the Nintendo and play for hours – or, really, until Eric can't keep his eyes open any longer. I remember those days.

Later at night, I'll stop by his room and take one of the comfortable window chairs. Jen sits next to me, her feet tucked underneath her legs, a red and white knit blanket covering her lap. Eric and I swap war stories about when we were first diagnosed. A sudden bolt out of nowhere for both of us, with similar symptoms that seemed like something else altogether. He hadn't bruised or bled nearly as much as me. I pull up my tee-shirt to show them the still-visible discoloration under my right arm and along the right side of my body from my first Hickman.

We talk about the Mariners, too.

He has also been a lifelong fan of our hard-luck professional baseball team. They've never had a winning record, never even had a whiff of a pennant race. It doesn't matter. This year — like every other year— we're convinced that they'll *finally* get it together. Ken Griffey, Jr looks like the real deal after a brilliant rookie season. With him in the outfield, and Harold Reynolds, Omar Vizquel, and Edgar Martinez taking care of the infield, coupled with a better-than-average pitching staff, we're optimistic. We've learned over the years to temper our enthusiasm. There's no denying it, though, the future is bright with this team.

An amazing thing happens one Saturday night, when Eric's parents are in town. Near the end of an otherwise uneventful evening, while the M's were playing a meaningless early season game against the Tigers, Randy Johnson throws the first no-hitter in franchise history! We watch replays and commentary on ESPN and the local news channels until well into the night.

We're both still giddy the entire next day. Scott comes over to visit in the early afternoon. Eric and his dad are already here, still watching highlights from yesterday, and the four of us spend hours talking about a game that none of us were able to attend. We reminisce about other memorable moments in our collective love affair with a mostly-mediocre hometown team: I'd been lucky one day, while at a game with Ian in high school, to have caught a baseball hit into the outfield. I was at the very edge of the seats and had to reach over with my mitt to catch the ball before it dropped into a wide gap below us. It was during batting practice, you know, so it didn't exactly count. But that official Major League Baseball still sits on my desk back at home.

Scott and I would usually try to get to the Kingdome for a game at least once or twice a summer. Indoor baseball isn't exactly the place you want to be during June or July in the summer. Eric and his dad agreed that they'd rather see games outdoors, but that didn't stop them from taking the long drive to Seattle once a summer since the Mariners first season – a family tradition that began when Eric and his younger brother were both in high school – regardless of who they were playing.

"Speaking of long drives," Eric's dad says, "your mother I and should get going. It's getting late. It's been a lot of fun, boys. Eric, we'll see you and Jen next week."

Scott says "I'm out, too. It's been great."

I thank all of them for their company as they make their way out of my room. It's been a great afternoon. These are good times. Surprisingly, incredibly, we've been able to *enjoy* our time in this place. It's hard to stop smiling about how good of a day it's been.

Anne walks through my door. I hadn't noticed how much time had passed. It's already the start of her shift: time for a quick check of my vitals. I'm giddy and exuberant, practically gushing about the amazing day, Randy Johnson's no-hitter, just everything being all kinds of awesome.

"*Awesome*," she says, almost under her breath.

She reaches out to check my pulse. It's immediately obvious that something's wrong. I've never seen Anne this quiet about anything. I ask her if everything is okay.

"Shh. Don't. Now I need to start over."

She lifts her fingers up from my wrist and then sets them back down again. Some number of seconds later she takes her hand away and writes something down. She reaches behind my head for the blood pressure cuff and wraps it around my arm. Before I can say anything else, she's already put a thermometer under my tongue. She's multi-tasking. Cuff unwraps. Little blue box connected to the thermometer beeps three times. Anne takes the thermometer out of my mouth.

"Is everything okay?" I ask again.

She takes a deep breath. "Yes. I'm sorry. It's been a bad start to the day. I really can't get into too many details other than to say that I lost a patient overnight."

"I'm…"

"It's okay, Robert. It happens. I'm just sad is all."

Of course it happens. I feel like an idiot. You don't get into nursing — especially oncology nursing — thinking that everyone you meet is going to pull through. This is the first time since I've been here, all absorbed with my own issues, my own problems, that it occurs to me that Cindy and Anne might have to work their way through bad days, too. *Of course* they're going to deal with death on a fairly regular basis. This is the cancer ward, after all.

"I'm sorry," I say.

"Thank you," she says, changing out the empty bag of antibiotics at the top of my cart.

I don't know what else to say.

* * *

I have a fair handle on the process by now. We'll use the factory analogy again, here, because Dr. Collins uses it often with me. And it's pretty accurate: your bone marrow is like a factory, producing all of these many different types of blood cells. It's amazing, and efficient, and resilient, the way the marrow keeps plugging away, creating healthy blood cells to send off into your bloodstream to do the good, important work that they need to do.

At some point, for some unknown reason, something goes wrong within the factory. Genetic mutation, maybe? 15;17 translocation? One of the production lines starts shipping immature, incomplete, not-ready-for-prime time blood cells. Platelets, let's say, hypothetically. The workers on that line don't know any better, necessarily, they just keep cranking out batch after batch of platelets that don't meet plant standards. They'd fail quality control. They do not work the way they are supposed to. But by the time anybody notices what's going on, it's been going wrong for far too long.

Chemotherapy is about shutting down the factory. Shut down the whole damn thing — even the production lines that didn't have any issues — and trust that management knows how to sort things out so that the factory can eventually resume production again.

Sometimes, unfortunately, it's not enough to just shut down the factory. Here's where a bone marrow transplant comes in: you need to nuke the first factory. Level it. Tear it to the ground. And then you replace it with another, hopefully identical factory, recognizing that only a wholesale change will be enough for healthy blood cells to start coming off that line again.

That I never needed a bone marrow transplant, Dr. Collins tells me, doesn't mean that we should forget about it entirely. She's being very helpful, really, spending so much time in my room, explaining things that I can't get my head around. Eric helps fill in additional context when I pester him with my questions. He knows much more about what a bone marrow transplant will look like than I do.

It's near the end of my consolidation round of chemotherapy. It's been too easy. Nice and perfect and on schedule, no complications. Like a walk in the park, if that park meant that you'd get chemicals meant to prevent your body from manufacturing any blood cells, while you sat around and watched movies and chatted with other patients and slept and had nurses and doctors tend to your needs. You know, that kind of a park.

And because my body has responded well, bouncing back when it's supposed to bounce back, Dr. Collins tells me that my bone marrow is the picture of health. There's another round of chemo on the horizon, consolidation again, sometime next month. I guess she's trying to tell me that I'm really *really* in remission now.

"But ..." I interrupt her. I'm used to this. The rosy picture is painted, but then reality has to set in. What is the "but" this time?

"But we can't *predict* a relapse, Robert. You are in remission. That is exactly where we'd hoped you'd be. If this round of chemotherapy doesn't stick, or even the one next month, we want to make sure we have other treatment options for you."

"I get that. There's no match in the registry for me, though, right?"

"True. There's no match *yet*. That's why we've scheduled a bone marrow harvest for you in a few weeks. In case you relapse, you'll be able to donate marrow to yourself."

The principle is sound: right now, I am healthy and cancer free. And my *own* bone marrow, should I ever need to receive a transplant, would be the best possible match. Far better than any random donor. More perfect than perfect, because it's mine coming right back.

The plan, then, is for me to go through that first stage of a transplant that Eric's younger brother will also be doing soon: harvesting the marrow from the donor. Instead of rushing that precious cargo off to a hospital, though, it will be saved somewhere in the bowels of the Fred Hutchinson Cancer Research Center. The phrase "put it on ice" comes to mind. I'm sure it's somewhat more complicated than a freezer filled with plastic containers of bone marrow, like leftover lunches at the office, my name and date scrawled on the top with a Sharpie. However Fred Hutch plans to store it, my marrow will be there for me if I ever need it again.

One of the shitty things about leukemia — one of many shitty things about cancers, in general, and their tendency to mutate and adapt — is that often the treatment that got you into remission in the first place is no longer effective after a relapse. As effective as my chemo has been, it's possible that a relapse would result in chemo being dramatically less effective, maybe even completely ineffective.

Often, especially with relapsed leukemia patients, there aren't any good options. It helps to be able to keep the possibility of a bone marrow transplant in our back pocket.

I love the idea of this insurance policy. As much as I don't like the idea that I might relapse, the simple truth is that it happens more often than it should. If I'm at a checkup in a few years and my new doctors are quietly shaking their heads as they look at my blood counts, telling me things I'd probably already know well before the blood draw — if that day comes, then we won't even need to go searching the donor rolls at the National Marrow Registry. I would be able to help myself.

✳ ✳ ✳

I've marked off 28 days on my wall calendar. One month exactly. It's Sunday, June 10th, and I'm going home again. I could not have predicted it would be like this, an exceptionally easy four weeks of hospitalization. Remarkably fun, even.

There were no unexpected complications, maybe one or two fevers that weren't particularly noteworthy, I didn't lose any weight because my appetite was mostly fine throughout. My muscles haven't atrophied like before. If anything, I feel even better and stronger today than when I'd arrived last month. That's unusual. That is not the normal course of chemotherapy, at least not compared with the last time I was in here.

The timing was absolutely perfect. It was exactly what Dr. Collins had described before we'd started: seven days of chemotherapy followed by twenty-one days of recovery. My counts had dropped to zero, as expected, and we had the appropriate responses lined up for everything. It was as close to perfect as we could have hoped for.

I'm excited to get out of here. Most of my friends are done with classes and finals by now, so I know there will be even more time to spend every day with them. Not entirely sure how long I'll have at home. When am I supposed to come back for my final round of chemo? A month, maybe? Sounds about right.

Figure a month at home, a month here again, and that will give me just about another month to get ready to go back to Carleton for fall term. Three months down, three to go.

Mom and Laura are here to pick me up. They've taken my things down to Mom's car and have left me to double check that I'm not forgetting anything. I want to stop by next door before I go. It's been getting tougher for Eric this past week. I feel for him. I think it's either today or tomorrow that he'll have been off his chemo for a full week, and for me, at least, it was that week when things got progressively worse. That's when it really hits you. He has another biopsy coming up soon to confirm that he's in remission.

I'd imagine that he won't be here when I come back later in the summer. Once he's in remission, his brother will drive or fly out from Spokane, and will go through the same process Dr. Collins had described to me for my own bone marrow harvest. Eric will have already been transferred to some kind of ultra-clean room at Fred Hutchinson where he'll both receive and recover from the transplant. Depends on a lot of factors, though, and I should know better than anyone that inducing remission via chemotherapy can take longer than expected. I'm honestly not sure when I'm going to see him again and I want to say goodbye while I can.

His door is slightly ajar. I knock once or twice, lightly, before walking in. Jen is napping in the chair next to his bed. He looks like he'd been napping, too, but his eyes are open when I peek my head into his room.

I'm dressed to leave. Shorts, shoes, sunglasses. No little buddy in tow. It feels liberating to be disconnected from all my meds. Eric starts to get up, but I'm quickly over by the open side of his bed, shaking my head, whispering for him to just stay put.

"I'm going home today," I say. "Kick ass, brother. You've got this."

"Thanks, man. You, too," Eric says.

"And stay in touch, okay?"

"Yeah. Definitely."

"Good luck with everything. With your transplant. Say 'goodbye' to Jen for me?"

He nods, then reaches over to rest his hand on his wife's shoulder. He pulls the light blanket up to his chin.

"See you," Eric says before his eyes flutter closed to continue his nap.

I try to be as quiet as I can, closing Eric's door behind me on the way out. I take the elevator downstairs. I'm dancing by myself in the empty elevator, shoulders quietly shimmying side-to-side, fists and arms close to my chest then wide open as I spin once, twice, smiling, shouting "yes!" to the emptiness. I'm free. I'm *out*. A beautiful Seattle summer awaits.

CHAPTER 28

There is a beautiful simplicity to my days at home. I've been working out. Riding my bike, running, doing push-ups and sit-ups like crazy, creating a makeshift gym in our living room after everybody's gone to sleep. I stay up late, watching TV, doing concentration curls and triceps extensions and shoulder shrugs. Then I tell myself to drop and give me twenty, gritting my teeth, elbows wobbling, swearing.

You fucking cancer, I say. You're not going to win.

Scott and I play fungo at Lindbergh. The wooden bat is the best, because it's more realistic, the crack of the bat. One of us stands at home plate, a half-dozen baseballs scattered around the backstop behind us. The other is in right-center, where the fence is closer. We try to knock the ball over the short fence. Lob the pitch up, then grip the bat with both hands, foot up, step into the swing. *Crack!* It's best if it's not a ground ball. You want the hard drive to right-center. You want to make Scott run, to pedal backwards to the warning track and watch the ball sail over the fence, bounce hard and high on the road just beyond, then scatter into the woods to be lost forever. It's worth buying a new ball at Toys-R-Us if you can hit the home run with the wooden bat.

The aluminum bat travels with us in the trunk of Scott's car, and we even bring it out with us when we hit balls and shag fly balls on sunny summer days. It's a lot easier to carry the fence when you're using aluminum, but it *pings*. A ping is not the crack of the bat. You have to *earn* those home runs with the wooden bat.

When we're not chasing down baseballs at the high school baseball field, then we're smacking golf balls into houses when we mean to hit fairways. Pitching and putting, spending hours in the sun. Or we're playing hoops at the courts near Tiffany Park. Scott's never afraid to put his body into it, under the hoop, banging me out of the way to get his own rebounds. He's always been much better than me at basketball.

"Take it easy," I tell him. He's bigger than me, has always used a strategy of pushing me around on the court, backing down, shoving me aside for relatively easy scores. And even though I've put some of the weight back on, I'm still rail thin. If I had a tough time beating him normally, it's even that much more difficult now.

Scott laughs at me when I complain. "Bulk up," he says. "Put on some weight! Do what you need to do. You don't get any gimmes in this game."

No gimmes, no pity. *Perfect.* It's just what I need.

Blake and I play tennis. There are a couple of courts at Coulon Park at the south end of Lake Washington. I try to make him run. I'm this lean, mean, can't hit a backhand machine, trying to speed my way to victory. It's so easy to get winded, though. I don't have much stamina. So I take a break on a dark green bench at the side of the court, smiling at the beauty of it all. I'm outside, spending time with my friends, working my legs.

This kind of medicine is essential. I drink it all in. They are fucking gorgeous, these summer days. The sun is brilliant and bright coming off the lake. Every day is a gift. I love them all.

Mom worries that I might pull out my Hickman. She tells me to just take it easy. I tell her that I've had months of taking it easy, and that I need to be stronger, still, for the third round that's yet to come. I need all my strength, I tell her.

In order to make sure my tennis racquet — or the golf club, or the bowling ball, or the frisbee — won't catch the two ports dangling from my right chest, I tape them to my stomach with strips of white tape. When I'm wearing a tank top, you can't even tell it's there. I don't take my shirt off, even at Coulon, with the water so cool and inviting. I'll wear a white tank top with my blue Carleton shorts. It'll be hot, and I'll be drenched in sweat, but I don't care. It's just so great to be outside, out of bed, getting stronger every day.

I eat often, sleep often. I run or lift during the days while my family and friends are at work or school. In the late afternoon there will be golf courses or kayaks or backyard barbecues. The stress melts from all of us. On weekends we drive downtown. I'm in the back seat and sometimes I'm more tired than I'm willing to let on, before the night has even started, and I'll let my head rest against the window. Scott will be driving all of us. He lights up a cigarette and reaches into the back seat to offer me one.

It's a joke we've stumbled across this summer, when he'll ask if I want a smoke, too. Sometimes he'll keep after it multiple times a night, because it's still so funny. He's being polite. That's what you do when you're out with your buddies, sharing your smokes. I'll decline every time because, you know, *cancer kid.*

I love these nights. We'll make it to Pioneer Square and stop to visit with Steckler, bartending at Casa de la Renaissance. He won't give us free drinks, but they'll be strong. I'll flirt with the cute bartender he works with and end up nowhere.

We end up at Doc Maynard's, Scott, Blake, Jeff and me. It's still relatively early, because these summer nights in downtown Seattle will sometimes find us out and about until one o'clock in the morning, if not later. One in the morning is a good stopping point, a natural break that allows us time to pile into Scotty's beloved Plymouth Horizon — the trusty steed that managed to drive several of us down I-5 to San Diego on an end-of-the-summer road trip the previous summer — and get to one of two Dick's Drive-In's before they close up for the night. A Dick's Deluxe, opened on the dash to add extra ketchup, with another couple two or three waiting in the bag, is always a great way to finish a night downtown.

So it's maybe midnight by the time we get to Doc Maynard's. I'm so happy, now, to have enough energy to be out and about this late. It hasn't even been a few weeks since I'd left the U, and no more than a week or so before I'll need to go back for more chemo, but all that is past and future. Tonight is about the present. About being present.

There are a couple of pool tables and dart boards in a back room, just a little bit beyond the main bar. Blake and I weave our way through the crowd while Scott and Jeff line up at the bar to get drinks for everybody. Pool tables, not surprisingly, are all being used. But there's an open board for darts. I drop some quarters in. Blake grabs a tall table near the window. It's raining again, just barely, and the streetlights outside catch the reflections on the wet pavement. I bring the darts back to the table and hand them to Blake.

"You're up first," I say. "Whenever the beer finally gets here, I mean."

We'll need the glasses for counter-balance. Darts in the right hand, a beer in the left, and the game feels much, much better. We both turn to look into the bar to see if Scott and Jeff have made any progress. A group of three girls at the next table over catch our eye. Sorority sisters, probably, or maybe a bunch of co-workers out for a night on the town. One blonde, and two brunettes. They're sipping from giant margarita glasses, laughing, looking over at Blake and me.

It's so easy for me to forget. I know what I look like, but it's still so easy to forget on these summer nights, where all I care about is quality time with good friends. I should know better by now. And now the blonde has stepped over to our table. She carefully sets her margarita on our table. It's strawberry—and worse, frozen, not on the rocks. I try not to judge.

"Hey," she says. Blake's big smile follows: not quite as much wattage as Scott's, but always pretty damn impressive.

"Hello," he says, reaching his hand across the table. "I'm Blake."

She makes eye contact with me. She ignores Blake's outstretched hand, instead bringing her free hand towards me, and suddenly I'm Mr. Shy, Mr. Awkward.

"Do you mind?" she asks me. "It's just that, well, I've never... Can I?"

Before I have a chance to answer, she's placed her hand on my head, softly bringing it back toward my neck, then up again. Is it my imagination? How did this cute blonde become infinitely more attractive? The touch of her hand is electric.

"What happened?" she asks.

Scott and Jeff materialize behind me, a tall glass of Red Hook in each of their hands, one for each of us. A quick exchange of heys and hellos while beers are distributed evenly, darts are scooped up from the table, and suddenly I'm alone with the cute blonde.

"So?" she asks again. "What happened?"

Decision time. What to do? What to say? It's so different, talking about leukemia with complete strangers. I'm not anywhere close to being done with this yet, okay, just taking time to live my life in between visits to the hospital. And I've already had way too many of these interactions where I end up feeling like I'm some kind of priest at a confessional, helping people receive some kind of absolution because they see that their lives — no matter how fucked up — couldn't possibly be worse than mine.

Friday night small talk becomes more difficult when the cute girl you want to chat up asks about the reasons why you don't have any hair. The truth is important, though, isn't it? I know it's easier to lie. I've gotten really good at it by now. But maybe she had a little brother with leukemia, or is studying nursing at the U. You never can tell with people. What if this is the beginning of the story of our future together? Meet cute at a crowded bar in Seattle, then marriage and babies and happily ever after. It's probably best to start with the truth.

"I have leukemia," I tell her. "I mean, I had it. Used to have it. I don't have it anymore. This is from the chemo. It'll grow back, though."

"Leukemia?" she asks.

"Yes. It's all right, though. I'm all better, now. Mostly all better, at least, just need one more round of chemotherapy and then I'll be good to go."

"Oh," she says. She sounds disappointed.

She smiles, wraps both hands around her jumbo-sized margarita glass, and takes a pretty little sip. She stands up to leave. "That's nice and all. I mean, you're cute, but you might want to come up with a better story. You should tell people you're in the Marines or something. I think that would sound better."

CHAPTER 29

A couple of days before the long Fourth of July weekend, I will come back to the hospital. Mom or Laura will drop me off in the morning. It'll be cool. Overcast. I'll make my way back up to the sixth floor. There is a somewhat hidden elevator bank that's reserved for patients — more of an express ride — and I hesitate for a minute before deciding to go ahead and use it. They have padded walls, a floor-to-ceiling grey padding, almost like a quilt, with enough room to fit a stretcher and several other people. It's the same way I'd arrived back in March.

The procedure is fairly simple, this bone marrow harvest. In fact, you could almost say that I've already had it performed on me, several times, only on a much smaller scale.

My first bone marrow aspiration – in that small, dark hospital room in Lancaster – feels so long ago. But it's only been about four months since Dr. Gorst first showed me the hollow needle that he would push into my bone. He'd needed a sample. My doctors here at the UW have needed samples, too, and they have used similar needles, pressing into my lower back. You don't need much marrow to do the kinds of tests that determine whether or not you have leukemia.

Again: same basic procedure, but with a few changes due to how much marrow needs to be retrieved from my body. Instead of a "little bee-sting, here," with a local anesthesia to numb my back, I will slowly count backwards from one hundred while a nurse pushes a needle of something into my Hickman Catheter. I won't make it past ninety-two before I'm out for the count. No need to be awake for this particular procedure.

And unlike my earlier bone marrow biopsies, which consisted of a single needing pushing into bone, it will be several. Or if not several needles, at least the one will need to be inserted several times into my bone. Did I say several? It's probably going to be closer to twenty or thirty separate extractions that Dr. Collins will need to make, in order to get enough marrow to send off to Fred Hutchinson. She will focus her efforts on two areas on either side of my lower back. Let's say ten to fifteen pokes on the left side, dotting a small circle, almost like a clock face, before switching over to do the same to my right. She needs enough marrow to get about a pint.

I'll wake up in the hospital sometime later in the afternoon. My back, not surprisingly, will be tender and sore. Like somebody whacked it repeatedly with a wood mallet. Or punched a bunch of holes into it with a long, hollow needle while I was sleeping.

There's a machine next to my bed that controls the intake of morphine into my Hickman. There's a button that I can push to get more. As much as I want, within reason. My back is sore. I should only be here for the rest of the day, maybe one more, tops.

Anne and I are talking about people who register, and are called on to donate marrow, but decline. It doesn't happen often, she tells me, but it does. I'm not going to lie: my back hurts like fuck. The aftereffects of the bone marrow harvest are easily in the top three of my most painful moments of the entire summer. And those other two — my first biopsy from Dr. Gorst, and my first Hickman from Dr. Hickman — probably hurt so much because of the shock and sudden new world I'd been thrown into. This is pain literally deep within my bones. I get that different people have different perspectives, and any number of reasons they wouldn't want to experience what this feels like. But I'm lying here doped up on all of this morphine and I can picture what it would mean to future me in a handful of years if all of my other options had run out and the only chance I had at survival meant that fit and tan and rested me had to deal with this pain for a few days. It makes me sad to think about. Why wouldn't you donate your bone marrow if you knew it could save a life? Pain fades into the background. It always does. Having my bone marrow harvested creates possibilities for the future. It's worth it.

Anne comes in to check on me when I can't figure out why the morphine machine doesn't work. She says it's because I've already taken too much. There's a limit. I tell her that I don't believe her and that my butt really hurts and could she please give me a butt massage.

That's how my smart, morphine-addled brain works. *Smooth.*

* * *

A few days later, back at home, Mom and I quietly load a few things into the trunk of her car in the early morning light. Dr. Collins wants us to be there by 8:00 so I can get started on my chemo, so Mom wants to make sure we're there by 7:30. Can't be late.

I'm wearing shorts and a tee-shirt. Pretty standard fare for most of the past month. God, I've loved this summer. I've gained back most of the weight I'd lost earlier in the year. I haven't felt this strong, physically, since well before February. I've been lifting and running and eating well and getting push-ups and sit-ups at nearly every opportunity. It's been absolutely glorious.

It's strange, I know, but I've been looking forward to getting back to see everyone again. This is the great thing about heading up to the UW for the third time this spring and summer. I know what to expect. The toughest part of this, everyone has agreed, was those first weeks. Induction. When my body was already so battered and bruised before our flight landed in Seattle. My counts were so dangerously low. I didn't know what to expect, then, but I got through the worst of it.

I've missed Cindy and Anne.

I used to feel like this when I'd pack for my annual month of summer camp at Camp Orkila. At first I'd be scared and nervous, worried about this strange new place that I'd only ever heard about from when Laura went there for a week by herself. After that first summer spent there, though, pretty much the entire month of July — not far off what I'm prepping for now — I absolutely fell in love. I couldn't wait to get back.

My nervous energy this morning, checking and double-checking I have everything I need — as if forgetting a book or a pair of pajamas would be the end of the world — is the same way I'd felt in my early teens on the night before my return to Orkila. There were good people waiting there for me. And I'd always very much looked forward to that.

Mom's nervous energy, on the other hand, as evidenced by the countless times she'd checked in on me while I'd packed, just to make sure everything's okay? She's obviously not thinking this is anything like bringing me to summer camp again. This isn't dropping me off in the parking lot at Northgate Mall to get on one of several busses filled with kids headed up to Orcas Island. It's not even close. This will arguably be the most difficult dose of chemo I've yet to receive, according to Dr. Collins. Mom is shouldering enough worry for the both of us, even though she's doing her best to hide it.

There's a little bit of traffic, but nothing terrible. We're going to be back at the hospital well before 7:30 at this rate. That's fine. I didn't sleep well last night — more nervous excitement — and I don't have anything planned for the rest of the day other than settling into a new but familiar routine.

We pull into the underground parking garage next to the University of Washington Medical Center. I've only been here a few times, but Mom knows exactly where to drive. It's a practiced maneuver into a corner space. This has been her routine. In the tunnel between the parking garage and the main hospital building, there's a long row of planter boxes along one of the walls — the right wall, as we're walking in — that have some gorgeous wildflowers brightening the passageway. I don't think I've ever noticed these before. Again, I've only been in and out of the parking lot a few times, but I would have expected to have at least noticed these flowers. They're spectacular!

I mention something about the flowers to Mom.

"Oh, yes," she says. "I noticed those straight away when Paul and I came in, the first day after you and I had come back from London. They were tulips then."

"It's nice," I tell her. "I mean, it's nice to have something pretty like this on the way into the hospital. I like that they do this."

"Yes," she says. "It is very nice. I've wondered how many different types of flowers I might see here before you get well. I said that to Paul on that first day. It's was tulips then, and it's something different now."

CHAPTER 30

indy is at the front desk when Mom and I come out from the elevators. She's as happy to see me as I am to see her. She dashes out from behind the desk to meet me with a hug before we're even halfway there. I'm all smiles.

She asks about our 4th of July holiday.

"It was sore," I say, rubbing both hands at the small of my back.

"Oh, that's right! Your harvest. Anne told me about *that*." We both laugh.

It really feels like a kind of homecoming. Scott and Blake and I have talked about this a couple of times over the past month or so, usually late into the night when we maybe start getting a little more serious about things. This concept of the "new normal."

See, the thing is that you can't really talk about the new normal without acknowledging things are different and really fucked up and we're all just adjusting to life around all of that. Because part of the new normal is skating along. It's not like we're pretending that everything is great when it's not. This has been an absolutely spectacular summer, and I have loved practically every minute of it. Elephant in the room, though, right? Leukemia? That thing that can still kill you even though you're in remission? Yeah. We don't talk much about that part.

The new normal, then, also applies here and now. It's why I am so ridiculously, unbelievably happy to be walking with Cindy to my new room. We're laughing. Telling jokes. I am so ready for this. One last week of chemo, some side effects that I've weathered before, a lot of spare time to read and write and play video games. Simple. I'll be back to Carleton in a couple of months, and life will move forward.

"You'll be on the other side again," Cindy says, referring to the far side of the wing, with windows facing west instead of east. Sunsets instead of sunrises, which is fine by me.

"Is Eric still there, too?" I ask. "Or is he already at Fred Hutch for his bone marrow transplant?"

Cindy stops.

"He's … no. I'm sorry, Robert. He never made into remission. His doctors were looking at options when pneumonia set in. This was a couple of weeks ago. He didn't make it. I'm so sorry. I thought you knew."

"He what?"

"I'm sorry," Cindy says again.

"That can't be right," I tell her. I'm struggling to figure this out. It doesn't make any sense. He was just *here*. And it's not as if we were best friends, lifelong buddies, I get that. I understand that. But we were warriors together. Twenty-somethings with the rest of our lives ahead of each other, ready to beat our respective diseases. It's not right. I'm sad and stunned and suddenly crying for somebody I barely knew.

Cindy takes me in her arms. She hugs me tight. "I'm so sorry," she says.

This is the part we don't talk about. That fucking elephant in the room looms large for a reason. Because this is normal. *This is expected.* This is the natural ebb and flow of things here on this floor that I'm so happy to have returned to. Cancer kills!

My friends and I haven't spoken those words out loud once this summer, but we've always known that's exactly what it does.

It doesn't take long to settle into my new room, just a few doors down the hall from where I'd been last month. My weights are in the corner underneath a purple and blue speckled chair. Deodorant and a toothbrush and toothpaste are set up by my sink. I'd brought my calendar back again, pinned up on the corkboard like before, along with a few of my favorite "get well soon cards" I'd received earlier in the summer.

Cards and letters have slowed significantly. Not that I mind. It's just a noticeable difference from when I'd first arrived, when it was this sudden and horrific news. Now that we've all settled into this pattern — especially with my friends here who have been out with me all summer, seeing me getting stronger with each passing day — it's almost as if I'm not sick anymore. I mean, I am in remission, after all. I've beaten cancer. That I need to spend another four weeks in this room before getting back to Carleton in September isn't that big of a deal. I've also brought a shoe box filled with more cards and letters that I've received since this all began. It's nice to have those kind words here with me.

Cindy has already brought in my medical cart — my little buddy — even though there's nothing on it yet. She'd done a quick check of my vitals, had asked me to take off my shirt so she could make sure my Hickman line was clean and accessible. She'll be bringing in my chemo in a bit, but Dr. Collins wants to explain it to us first. This will be a little different, this final round, so we're waiting for the good doctor, my excellent primary oncologist, to arrive with her patient explanations.

Mom has brought one of the window chairs up alongside my bed again. I'm pacing around the room, not ready to claim the bed just yet.

I'm still mad about Eric.

Mom has already said "I'm sorry" a few times in the short time since Cindy told me what happened. I know she means well. I'm also sure that she doesn't want to dwell on the obvious. Neither do I. That doesn't make me any less angry about a stupid fucking disease that arbitrarily picks and chooses victims. Eric and I were both young. Both strong. Both healthy, aside from the leukemia. We both had the same nurses and the same doctors and the same strong support network. His wife, Jen, was always with him, every time I'd stopped in to visit. Eric was optimistic. He had a much stronger faith in God than I've ever had — summers spent at a YMCA camp shaped my spiritual beliefs toward the outdoors, toward nature, instead of organized religion within a church. Not Eric. His faith was strong.

Eric had everything going for him. It just doesn't make any sense. And that's put me into a sour mood well before Dr. Collins finally comes through the door with her ever-present clipboard and white lab coat.

It's good to see her. I'm happy to see her, of course, just as I was with Cindy, just as I know I will be when Anne comes into work later this afternoon. But I'm fuming. I've sworn at cancer a lot over the summer. When I'm trying to get that one last rep in or pushing myself to run to the top of a painful hill, I've often sworn at cancer under my breath. For the first time, though, I hear myself thinking the words "it's not fair."

Dr. Collins is all business. She's not rude or insensitive. She's here to speak with me about this next month of treatment, though, not counsel me on the loss of a friend on a floor where death visits regularly.

She greets me first, then my mother, only minimal small talk about the past few weeks, my bone marrow harvest, and a "nice summer we're having here" before she asks me if I remember our earlier conversations about what this round might look like. She doesn't mention Eric. Now is not the time to be reminded of my mortality.

She'd taken some extra time at the end of one her rounds, way back in April, to sketch out our long-term goals. We'd made it through the worst of it by then. Dr. Collins knew that this wouldn't be enough. She knew that we'd also need some longer-term treatment plans. When you're dealing with leukemia, "long-term" gets friendly air-quotes. It means getting me through the rest of the summer not the rest of my life. We'd known, then, that our most important priority was remission.

"Induction," she'd told us in April, "is what we're doing now. Induction therapy: *inducing* remission, as it were." She'd gone on to explain that in order to give me the best chance for long-term success that I'd need two additional visits to the hospital for two additional weeks of chemo known as "consolidation therapy." She'd said it was as if we'd painted a room in my house: induction therapy was the primer, but we'd still need two more coats of paint on top of that to make sure the job was done right.

I'm about to tell Dr. Collins that I remember what she'd said about needing a couple of extra coats of paint when Mom chimes in.

"You'd said this one was going to be different than first two times Robert was here. Similar, but different?"

Dr. Collins smiles wryly. "Yes, that's right."

"How so?" I ask. I don't remember this part.

She smiles again, tapping at one of the empty hooks on my "little buddy."

"The main difference, Robert, is what we'll be putting up here for you. You're much stronger now. Much healthier. You've been doing a great job with rest and recovery. Because of that, we want to hit your leukemia harder now than we have before. Hit it hard while it's on the run. The most effective way to do that is to move away from the 7+3 protocol we've used so far. We're going to eliminate the seven days of ara-C and bump up the intensity and potentially the duration of the daunorubicin."

"Bump up the intensity? Seriously? I thought it already *was* pretty intense. That's why I only got it for three days at the end of each week?"

"Yes. You're right. This is a significantly stronger version, though, a high-dose daunorubicin. It's much stronger. Like you."

"Still just the three days, then?"

"Well," she says. "At *least* three days. It's best for you to receive this for a full seven days, similar to what we did before. It's going to be difficult, I know, since this is more potent than anything you've received yet. I need you to get as close to that week as you can. I need to give you this chemo for as long as your body can take it."

I nod in agreement.

Fuck you, cancer, and what you did to Eric. Bring it on.

CHAPTER 31

This week passes by in a blur. So much of it is the same as it ever was — Cindy brings my new chemo in before Dr. Collins has finished talking with Mom and I about the ramifications of a much stronger dose.

It looks pretty much the same as before. The steady drip commences. Mom and I talk through my plans for the fall. I am trying to move past the past and am so looking forward to getting back to Carleton. I'd made certain, before this last round of chemo, to write and send all the final essays I'd needed to pass my classes in Lancaster. My professors there had been more than lenient with me, asking me to only tackle the final essay instead of all the other assignments I'd missed due to my hasty departure from the University there. At the very least, then, I won't be missing any credits when I return to school. I've still missed all of spring term at Carleton that will need to be made up somehow.

"You can cross that bridge when you come to it," Mom says.

"I know," I tell her. "It's hard to believe that I'll be back on campus in only a couple of months."

"Hopefully," she says. "Let's hope."

Lunch arrives on a beige trey. It's unremarkable. I'm not hungry but eat it anyway. Force of habit these days: when one *can* eat food, one always does.

Cindy comes in to check my vitals again, probably the last time today before her shift is done. I sit in one of the chairs while she does this. The bed can wait. I'm not sick yet. I want to stay out of that bed as much as I can.

Mom excuses herself to get a late lunch from the cafeteria. In that brief moment of privacy, I drop to the floor and work through several sets of push-ups and sit-ups and dumbbell curls, all of it careful and methodical to make sure I don't get caught up in any of the tubing connecting me to my little buddy. Mom returns from lunch with a small cup of coffee for each of us.

"I can only stay a little longer," she says. "Traffic starts to get bad so early."

Time passes. I know that Dad and Jane will be stopping by later this evening. Anne should be arriving soon, too, to start her shift. I escort Mom to the elevator, wheeling my little buddy alongside us. I want to get some more exercise anyway. Every little bit helps, just walking the length of the two main hallways that divide this floor, just a couple of quick laps. I avoid Eric's door.

This could be any day. This routine, this familiarity, this comfortable sense of belonging blends in with all the other days before and after it. And I know what's coming, too. There are no surprises at this stage. I'm a seasoned veteran, starting up my fourth week of chemo in about as many months. I know exactly what this chemo is going to do to my blood counts. Seven days of healing poison entering my body followed by three weeks of recovery. Simple. Clockwork.

Not to say that it's going to be easy. Of course not. No doubt I'll spike some crazy fevers again. That's nothing new. I seem to be particularly gifted at getting high fucking fevers, which we'll treat with a cycle of hot blankets and icy washcloths, a full array of antibiotics when my counts are down for the count, ultimately leaning on Demerol to cut the edge. My appetite will fade into nothingness at about the same time as my energy levels and enthusiasm for hospital hallway walks and hospital room workouts.

It will be the same as before. Scott visits. Blake visits. We'll talk about the Mariners, or we'll play video games, and it will be good. We'll skate around the new elephant in the room, that Eric is no longer here to share those moments.

Laura stops over for an hour or two after work, a few days each week, sometimes with Dad and Jane, sometimes with Mom and Paul. Sometimes my room will be crowded with friends and family and I'll get snappy with them as my energy levels continue to drop, then I'll feel bad about it afterward.

All of this is expected. It's all completely normal. Except it's not. There's something different about this chemo. I can't put my finger on it. Maybe it's just as simple as what Dr. Collins had said before we'd started: it's extremely potent. I can taste it almost immediately. I'm pretending like I can't, but it permeates *everything*. It isn't supposed to start fucking with my body this soon. The way it's supposed to work, the way it's felt every other time — you know, the whole two other times I've walked into this hospital to receive chemo — is this general malaise, this slow incremental build-up where I kinda sorta feel maybe a little lousier each day for a week. Appetite fades, remember? It doesn't just vanish. Energy levels should slowly taper instead of getting destroyed.

This week is not at all what I'd expected. This high-dose daunorubicin is *brutal*. As always, the fevers arrive first, like an old friend who hasn't visited in years. I can tell they're coming well before Anne checks my vitals. It's summer, but it shouldn't be this hot in the hospital room.

"One-oh-five," Anne says with some concern. "You doing okay? Do you want some hot blankets?"

I shake my head. "Too hot."

"I'll be right back," she says. I know she's off to get a new bag of antibiotics to put at the top of my cart. She'll come back with Tylenol, too, and probably a big bowl filled with ice and washcloths.

I'm always hot first. We work through this. We cool my forehead down with a rotating arsenal of washcloths, soaked in ice, squeezed mostly dry, wiping at my face and neck and shoulders while sweat drenches my tee-shirt.

I lose track of time. Minutes? Hours? Chills always follow, no matter what. I need to change out of my tee-shirt because now it's soaked with sweat and freezing, too, and my entire body begins to tremble and shake. Chattering teeth. Goosebumps everywhere.

This used to scare me in the early days. Now I know it's just my body working through current limitations. My immune system is compromised again. That's the price of admission. That's the path to wellness. Fevers are just the first familiar indicator that I'm struggling with these old rules of engagement again.

Anne brings in several piping hot blankets to bury me under. One blanket is never enough. She stacks several without checking if I want them or not. She knows. She knows how my fevers work. She tells me about the Demerol, shows it to me, swabs one of my free Hickman ports with a small square antiseptic wipe before the needle goes in. It'll help with the chills. It always does.

This is our routine. It's a process. This is how we work the problem. I'll be falling asleep soon. Demerol and other drugs, the warm blankets, the chemo-induced fatigue all conspire to push my fevers into the background. They might stay away for a few hours, maybe more, but I trust that they'll be back. It's okay. It's good. We're cool. We're buddies. They're oddly comforting, these fevers of mine, these regular reminders that my days here are not meant to be easy. Survival comes with costs.

Like nearly every other time I've been here, we start stacking up a variety of antibiotics to help combat my fevers. That's what happens when the chemotherapy has been effective in shutting down my bone marrow's production of healthy blood cells. I've got nothing left inside me that's going to be able to help fight infections — I'm neutropenic, again — so I'll be getting a little outside assistance.

For the most part, though, the antibiotics don't seem to be helping much. Dr. Collins prescribes some additional bags to add to the top of my cart, knowing that there will be some overlap with my existing antibiotics. It feels like we're kind of taking a "kitchen sink" approach this time, throwing everything we can at these fevers.

I've been getting low, dull headaches, pervasive, seemingly independent of the fevers. So we start up on a regular dose of Tylenol. Dr. Collins suggests adding even more antibiotics. I don't argue with her. She knows best, right? I can't keep track of how many different bags are on my cart now, some seemingly always full, some nearly depleted, all working together to address the same problem.

That's something else that's like nearly every other time I've been here: what Dr. Collins really wants is to find the source of my fevers. Where are they coming from? What's the root cause? Antibiotics, of course, are a tremendous help, but they don't get her any closer to understanding *why*. Same as before.

That's why she starts scheduling visits for me down in radiology again. It's time for more X-rays. I hope she finds what she's looking for. I don't even want to consider the possibility that we might have to chase them down with even more invasive procedures like another bronchoscopy. Or, worse, that she'll need to pull out my second Hickman. I'm hoping that X-rays are enough.

CHAPTER 32

I wake up to something new. Fevers have still been kicking my ass, and the dull headaches continue to throb. If I rest my head in my hands I'm able to feel my forehead pulsing against my palms. I've gotten used to these things. What's unusual this morning is the fact that my room is painfully bright.

I slide out of my bed and shuffle over to the light switch, eyelids squinched up tight, my free hand providing additional cover as if I'm walking into the morning sun. But the sun rises on the other side of the building, so that doesn't make any sense. I'm immediately frustrated that one of my overnight nurses — Kenna was last night, I think — must have left the lights on after she'd come in for vitals and to swap out one of many bags of antibiotics that have been growing at the top of my little buddy.

My hand slaps against the wall where the light switch should be. I want to get back to bed. That's weird: my lights are already turned off. *What the ...?*

If my lights are off, then why is it so bright in here? I shuffle over to the sink so I can take a look in the mirror, still shielding my eyes from the overhead lights that aren't even on. It's tough to open up my eyes enough to see because it's so fucking bright. But it's already obvious: my right eye is pinkish. Not much of any visible white to see, just an angry, irritated reddish pink eye.

Great, I mutter to myself. *Just what I need.*

I have a few questions about my eye for Dr. Collins when she comes in for her rounds. I've been keeping my eyes closed, kind of burying my face in my pillow while I wait for her to arrive. It helps makes the room even darker. My breakfast is on the cart at the end of my bed, untouched.

She has a few questions for me, too, one of which involves permission to use a small pen light she keeps clipped in a pocket on her lab coat.

"It hurts just to open my eyes without any lights on," I tell her.

"Yes," she says, "I know. But I need to take a look."

The pain is brief and excruciating. I have to hold my eyelids open with my right hand. They flutter against my fingers, trying to avoid the light. Dr. Collins performs only a cursory check, shining her light into my right eye, then my left, then my right again. Tears come almost instantly.

"I'm sorry," she says. She puts the pen light back in her pocket. She makes a few marks on her clipboard. "I'm done now. Is there anything else you've noticed? Anything else since last night? Other than the fevers, of course."

"No," I say. I'm trying to remember. "I still have a headache, but those have been coming and going for a while now."

"Yes, yes," she says. She writes something else down on her clipboard. "I'm going to schedule an appointment with one of our ophthalmologists here. I'd like to find an opening for later today. This doesn't look like pinkeye, Robert, and I want them to give you a proper examination. I'd also like to get you in for a CT scan

— a CAT scan — for your headaches. There are a lot of moving pieces for us to look at."

"Do you think they might be related? The headaches and fevers and everything?"

"We won't know until we get the results back. It's definitely an eye infection, though, not pinkeye, but I don't know enough about it yet to know if it's related to your fevers. Obviously with your neutropenia we're going to want to be extra cautious. Oh. Yes. That reminds me of something else I'd wanted to speak with you about this morning. Cindy reminded me that we've been giving you a lot of Demerol lately, yes?"

"Yeah. Whenever I get chills from my fevers. It helps."

"But not as much as it used to?"

I'm not sure. I'm thinking about the past couple of days, trying to remember if I've been getting fevers more often, or chills more often, or if the Demerol hasn't been knocking me out as quickly.

"I don't know," I say to Dr. Collins. "I guess I haven't really noticed."

"It's okay. We have. You've built up something of a tolerance for it, unfortunately, and I'm not comfortable increasing your dosage. In fact, I'm taking you off it altogether, effective immediately."

"What? *Why?*"

"The last thing you need right now is to be fighting an addiction, too. It's not been working as well, Robert. There are other alternatives we can use to help with your chills. I've already told the nursing staff. No more Demerol for you. I'm sorry."

✳ ✳ ✳

The thing about eye doctors is, you know, they need to look in your *eyes*. They need to shine a very bright light into each eye, one at a time, and then they need to do it again. They might give you something in a dropper, first, to help dilate your pupils, to provide additional information, or context.

They'll also want to take photos of your eyes. It's not just the one doctor, or the two or three, as the case may be, who are interested in the unusual infection that's caused significant inflammation, particularly in your right eye. It's a rare thing they're seeing, so they need to document it.

In other words, each of the trips that will be taken to the helpful, friendly, studious, concerned ophthalmologists will require much more time than you'd expected. More to the point: you've taken to wearing the black Ray Bans your sister had given to you for your birthday throughout the hospital, at all hours, because that at least allows you to squint your way through the painfully bright indoor lights. Your expectation, then, of how long you should have to spend with your chin resting on the padded edge of this monstrous torture machine is right around no minutes. Zero minutes at all would be perfect for these visits with the ophthalmologists.

I need to keep my eyelids pried open with my fingers. I can only do one at a time. We take breaks often. I alternate hands — one to keep whichever eye is being examined open, the other to hold a tissue I need for wiping the tears away. These are useful, important tests that will help us get to the root of things.

* * *

"They're related," Dr. Collins is telling us.

I'm where I feel like I always am when she has important news to tell me, sitting as upright as possible in bed. The problem is, of course, that whenever she has important things to say, I'm feeling particularly fucked up. Tonight is a fantastic combo platter of painfully sore eyes, my entire forehead throbbing with a jackhammer of a headache, a fever that's upwards of 105 again with no Demerol in sight, so I trust that I'll just have to ride out the chills when they stop by for a visit soon. I'm keeping my eyes closed, trying to hold a coldish washcloth on my forehead, clenching my jaws way too hard for all of this. That's not going to help.

I try to relax. It's hard. Mom and Paul and Dad and Jane are all here, all of us listening to Dr. Collins explain that, unlike the variety of tests and X-rays I'd had back during my first hospital stay, the CAT scan was a success. They've found a number of abscesses in my brain. The eye infections, my fevers, and obviously the headaches are all part of the same fundamental problem.

That's *success*, I guess? Fucking infections in my brain? Thanks, Dr. Collins.

I'm letting my parents steer the conversation. They have all the questions at the ready. I suppose this isn't really a surprise, is it? Leukemia works this way. Sneaky backstabbing mother fucker. And, really, at this point it's not even leukemia's fault, right? I don't have it anymore. I've been in remission for months.

Fuck. I'm splitting hairs now. It's been necessary for me to have this final round of chemotherapy in order to have a hope at long-term survival. I know this. I get this. I've welcomed this last round. I wanted to come back, wanted this chemo, wanted to feel comfortable with the knowledge that we were pulling out all the stops. Of course the blame for this still rests squarely on the shoulders of my leukemia. My body is more prone to infection when I don't have a functioning immune system. That's just the way it works. Luck of the draw. Brain infections.

I'm trying to unclench my entire upper body at this point, arms and shoulders and jaws all tense and tight, fighting through the onset of chills. It feels like somebody has swung an aluminum bat at my head. There's no *ping*, though, so it must be a nice wooden bat, instead.

God, I'm such a fucking mess. I couldn't even eat a bowl of dry cereal earlier. Not because of nausea, but because I was trying to eat with my eyes closed against the brightness of nothing and my arms were shaking so much, trembling, Demerol withdrawals maybe, and the Cheerios flew off the spoon before I could get them into my mouth. I eventually just dumped the bowl onto the tray and picked at them one at a time. Like a baby. Helpless.

I hear Dr. Collins say something about an MRI. I open my eyes a sliver, hoping that will help me pay more attention. The lights are off. It's still not dark enough. Dr. Collins is standing near my bed, next to my little buddy and the myriad bags of antibiotics on top of it. Apparently, I have an appointment to get an MRI in the morning.

"It's like a CAT scan," Dr. Collins says, "except it's 3D. The CAT scans show us that you have a number of abscesses that need to be treated. We just don't know exactly where they are."

"Why do you need to know that?" Dad asks.

"Yeah," I chime in. "What does it matter where they are?"

"Well — and this is why you'll be meeting with the neurologists tomorrow, too — we need to know more in order to effectively treat them. If one or more are close to the surface, it might be good to consider surgery as an option."

"Surgery?" Jane asks. "You're talking about brain surgery? That's significant."

"Yes. It's early yet. But you can see how many antibiotics we've been giving Robert, and they're just not enough. We need to know more."

* * *

It's not just the one MRI, which is almost immediately helpful. Three dimensional images are better, of course. Dr. Collins is never wrong. Turns out we need multiple scans, multiple images. We're building blueprints. The more accurate the blueprints, the better.

When one of the neurologists comes into my room with Dr. Collins later, so they can both explain what all of this means, I can't get past the arrogance. I'm sure he doesn't mean it, this talented, thin, bald doctor who smells of mints whenever I see him. It's not his fault that we're not really asking him to do anything challenging. He's not going into my head to fix anything. He's just going to take a sample.

Whatever good the constant cycle of antibiotics I'm on now is doing — and I'm sure those endless bags are working wonders — they're not preventing these crippling headaches, my worsened eyes, or the regular return of high fevers. That means we need to figure out what's happening in my head. And the only people who can do that for me don't exactly have a lot of bedside manner.

I'm downstairs again, tucked into this tiny claustrophobic tube, pinging noises all around. I've lost track of how many of these brain scans I've had recently. My surgery is coming up soon and, understandably, the doctors responsible for cutting a hole in my head want the most current information. I don't have any idea how abscesses work. Are they stationary? Do they settle into a favorite spot and just relax? Or do they grow, change, move around? Are these MRIs showing brain abscesses like continental drift? Is that why I'm down here multiple times a day?

And then I can feel chills coming on. Fucking fevers. *Fucking chills.* I can't control what happens when they come. My entire body tightens to try to stop from shaking but it doesn't do any good. The pinging stops. There's a muffled sound from the technician across the room, behind the glass.

"I need you to hold still, Robert. We need to get these images locked in. You're all over the place on us."

"I'm trying," I say. I *am*. Why doesn't anybody believe me?

Nothing works. Since Dr. Collins cut off my Demerol, nothing has worked to eliminate these fucking chills. It's just a storm I've had to learn to weather. They eventually pass. I *know* how important these MRIs are. I hate them, hate that incessant pinging, hate the pressing feeling of claustrophobia. You don't need to tell me twice why they're so critical.

I can't stop shaking.

"Let's just take a break," the tech says.

My eyes are closed tight. My cheeks are wet. I wish I could stop these chills. I wish I knew how to make them go away. I'm rolled out of the MRI. There's a familiar hand at my shoulder. I don't know how she knew to be here, but here she is.

"It's okay," Cindy says.

She covers me with a hot blanket. Two. Three. She takes a small vial and a needle from her pocket. "I asked Dr. Collins and she said it would be okay, just this once."

The Demerol is instantly effective. That push. That rush. Everything melts.

"It's going to be okay," Cindy says again, as I slide backwards into a dark metal tube. "You're going to be okay."

CHAPTER 33

I hate this floor. Literally, this stupid carpeted floor, with this faded brownish beige kind of artsy checkerboard pattern. And this entire hospital wing while we're at it, all of 6 SE. I hate how helpful and friendly the nursing staff are when I barely get one foot in front of the other on the way back to my room. We're in between shifts, now, and I don't recognize anybody. Why can't Cindy and Anne be here all the time? Stupid fucking staffing models. It's ridiculous, is what it is.

A nurse I don't know is at my side, helpful, concerned, offering an arm to get me the rest of the way to my room. "Or do you want a wheelchair?" she asks.

"No," I say. "*No!*" I can still walk. I'm not an invalid. I'm slow, and it's hard to see, but I don't need any help.

These fucking lights! I hate how bright they've become, even with my sunglasses on. I wish I didn't have to wear these sunglasses indoors in the first place. I know that's my fault, too: it's these eye infections that we've tracked back to the abscesses that my neurologists are so goddamn cavalier about.

All I want right now is to get back to my room, to close my door, and have some time to myself. Is that too much to ask? I know the answer before I even ask it: *Yes. Yes, of course it is.*

This is not a hotel. As much as I try to personalize it, my room is not mine. If it was, there'd be a lock on the door. A huge fucking deadbolt. I'd click my door shut, if I could, lock that deadbolt from the inside, push all the chairs and other furniture up against the door for good measure, just in case hospital security showed up with a crowbar. What a pipedream.

This is a hospital, not a hotel. In this world, my reality for months, a closed door simply means that my doctors and nurses *might* knock once or twice before pushing in anyway, apologetic, regardless of how I answer. I don't think they even wait for an answer these days. They might as well just take the door of the hinges. It might as well not even exist.

I hate it here. I hate everything about it. I hate these walls, these halls, these doors that can't lock. All of it. My room is still forever away from the front desk and all I want is to crawl into my bed and turn my back to a door that never keeps anyone out. I just want *everyone* to give me some space, some tiny measure of solitude for five fucking minutes. *Please.*

* * *

Blake visits, as usual. He's waiting in my room when I get back from yet another round of MRIs. It's so good to see him. I've been hating the MRIs more and more lately, and it's nice to have his consistent and comforting presence now that I'm back. It's been like this all spring and summer, with Blake and Scott and Jeff in particular, either here or at home: my friends have stuck with me. They have been at the ready to pick me up when I fall down. Physically, emotionally, whatever. I don't know how they do it. I don't know that I would have been able to do the same thing if I was in their shoes. They've kept me so grounded.

Even just the amazing simplicity of Blake's presence. We both know that we don't necessarily need to talk. Hell, I don't even have to stay awake! We might be watching a movie together, and I'll wake with a start. The TV will have been turned off and Blake will just be sitting in the room close to me. Sometimes he'll fall asleep, too. My best friends have been more supportive than I could have ever hoped for — appearing as if by magic when I sleep, staying by my side because they want to be here, not because I'd ever asked.

"Hey, buddy" he says, setting down the book he'd been reading while waiting for me.

I slowly make my way to the bed.

Fuck! Headaches are back with sudden fury. I just need to lie down. I cover my eyes with both hands, palms resting on my cheek bones. I've found this is the best way to keep things as dark as possible. I'm also able to keep my thumbs resting on both sides of my forehead, a gentle massage where these headaches usually feel the worst. I'm taking slow, deep breaths, trying to breathe through the immediacy of this pain.

"You doing okay?"

"What do you *think*, Blake? Does it look like I'm doing 'okay?'"

"I'm sorry, man. Headaches again?"

"Of course it's the headaches! What else could it be? Where did I just get back from? Seriously? That's all we ever do any more, scanning my brain twelve times a day because that one extra time is sure as shit gonna tell my doctors what they need to know to stop these abscesses from killing me!"

There's silence. I don't know why I'm so angry right now. I don't know why Blake is still here. So I ask him: "why are you here, Blake?"

"I'm sorry, RK. Do you need me to get Cindy to come take a look?"

"No! No, I don't. How do you think this is going to play out? Everybody knows what's happening. I'll be gone soon and you just don't want to feel guilty after that happens. *Why are you here, Blake?* Are you just punching the clock so you won't feel like such a shitty friend when I'm dead?"

My temples feel like they're exploding. Countless throbbing explosions perfectly synchronized on either side of my head. The noise is deafening. The room is shifting on me. Tilting.

I think I can hear Blake getting up from his chair. He still hasn't said anything. I take my hands away from my face and see him already at the door. He stops, briefly, on his way out.

"Fuck you," he says. Twice, maybe. I don't know. He doesn't bother to close the door behind him.

Cindy comes in a little while after Blake leaves. I'm not sure how much time has passed. It's like that again, like it was in the beginning, when it's so difficult for me to keep track of something as basic and fundamental as the time of day. It doesn't help that my head is still throbbing. Or that I've been caught in something of a loop, continuing to replay what I'd said to Blake, now regretting all of it.

Cindy has a workout bag over one shoulder. Her car keys jangle in her right hand. She tells me that her shift had finished earlier and she's on her way home now.

"I know when your shift ends," I tell her. "I've been here long enough to know."

"I just wanted to check in to see how you're feeling," she says.

There's genuine concern in her voice. She legitimately cares about me as a person, and as a friend. I know that I mean a lot to her. I *know* this. That doesn't stop me from telling her that she shouldn't have bothered. She should just go home already. I tell her that I know I'm just a number to her, just part of the job, that she doesn't need to pretend to care about me anymore.

She kind of half smiles, steps closer so she's standing right next to my bed, just as she's done countless times throughout the countless days that I've been stuck in this fucking hospital.

"You are going to get through this," she says. "I know you will." And then she turns and walks out, quickly, leaving me alone to keep feeling sorry for myself for another couple of hours, at least.

Anne arrives, later, to begin our evening routine of vitals and meds, swapping out empty bags of antibiotics for new ones. She takes my pulse. Puts the back of her hand against my forehead before reaching for the large blue thermometer on the wall behind me to get more precise measurements. Her hand is firm on my wrist.

"I know you're feeling off, Robert. I know you've been scared. But don't even *think* about starting up with me, too."

CHAPTER 34

Night falls. My room is quiet. It was quiet, too, earlier in the evening when Mom and Paul had visited briefly. I was all one-word responses to any of their questions, mostly "no," killing conversation in favor of watching a little TV together — the sounds from the television nothing more than steady white noise to block out the rest. I know they're worried about the surgery tomorrow. Mom in particular. Her body language is wound up, tight, tense while she keeps dancing from pleasant subject to pleasant subject. I just don't want to talk about *anything.*

But that's a different sort of quiet than what happens late at night, when I'm restless, and I've woken up from another fever-induced dream. They're vaguely unsettling, these dreams, that don't wake me suddenly. It's the opposite. It's as if I'm sliding into reality, beating open my eyes in the near darkness, the blurry outline of my room never really getting to sharp, not quite awake and not quite asleep, struggling to find my bearings. I can't focus on anything. I'm not blind but I still can't see.

I know it's because of the eye infections, and I know those are going to be treated, too, once my surgery determines exactly what these abscesses are doing inside my skull. I can process all of that just fine, my young logical mind, but it still doesn't change that deep uneasy feeling that's been lingering with me for the better part of a week now.

It would be great if I could get up and go for a walk. I'd be back to my old slow shuffle — head down, barely moving, leaning on my little buddy for support — and that would certainly help give me a bit of clarity. I can't, though. I wouldn't be able to *see*. It's as simple as that. It's too bright in these halls. I'm not about to don my sunglasses at night just to shuffle aimlessly in several rough circles through this floor filled with dying patients.

Because that's what I am, now, isn't it? A dying patient? One more statistic waiting to happen?

I hate what I'd said to Blake earlier. Hate how I'd treated Cindy. I wish I could take it back. The truth is a hard thing to face when you're all alone in a dark and silent hospital room. It's only me, now. I force myself up. Make my way over to the sink near my bed. Hands on the edge of the counter for support. I look in the mirror. I'm not looking to see how red and infected my eyes continue to be, or how gaunt and skeletal my face has become.

I need to look in the mirror. I mean, really look, for this one moment, maybe, and allow myself to admit a painful truth: I am scared to death of death.

And it's not only that fundamental fear that my days are markedly numbered that's keeping me awake. Let's assume that the surgery is successful, and my neurologists will soon have the necessary details about my brain abscesses so they can prescribe the perfect combination of antibiotics, which I will dutifully take for as long as they tell me to take them. *Fine.* But what if something happens when they open up my skull? It's my fucking *brain* they're touching. This will easily be the most invasive procedure I've had since I've been here.

My team of neurologists, bless them, will continue to treat it like the simple oil change that it is to them. They're used to working on Ferrari's, Lamborghini's, all sorts of complex and challenging surgeries through the pathways of our minds. Their supreme confidence — *overconfidence?* — doesn't make me feel any better. It might be the most routine of routine maintenance jobs to them, this dead simple task of drilling out a quarter-sized chunk of my skull to do nothing more than acquire a sample of the abscess that will be exposed directly underneath said hole in my head.

I get that. There's nothing routine about it for me, though. What if I'm standing in front of this mirror in a few days and I don't even recognize the person that I see? A wire could cross, right? Something could change. And I would be permanently, irrevocably, different. What if I'm about to become a completely different person and I won't know that I've changed? Or, worse, I do, but am unable to do anything about it? I'll be like a prisoner in my own mind, doing and saying things that I don't mean to do or say. My friends and family will all remember what I was like before, and wistfully think back on that much nicer, kinder, gentler version of me and say "we sure thought you were pretty great back then, but … at least you're still alive today."

Grandpa's favorite phrase comes to mind: *could be better, could be worse.*

Far too many times this month I've been reminded that the worst case isn't my theoretical post-surgery identity crisis, it's that I don't even make it to the operating table. It's been hard for me to rest this week partly because of those philosophical fears, but mostly, I think, because I've been afraid that any time I fall asleep might be my last. I don't dwell on it. I don't cross my fingers and say "hope to *not* die" at bedtime. But I have to be realistic about a few things and the reality of leukemia is that this is how it happens.

I've been exceptionally lucky. So crazy lucky it's not even funny, with how much I'd bled before I even left England. That was the real risk: bleeding to death, before I even had a chance to start chemotherapy. Luck doesn't last forever, though, does it? If leukemia is going to end me, this is probably how it's going to do it.

This, Grandpa, is your "could be worse." Brain infections kill. That's what they do. It was pneumonia for Eric. Why shouldn't it be this for me?

I'm staring at someone I can only assume is me in the mirror and I am absolutely sobbing. My body heaves. I grab a handful of tissues and try to blow my suddenly stuffed nose. It doesn't do any good. My cheeks are damp, tears roll down and off my chin, spittle coming out of my mouth when I try to breath. It hurts. Everything hurts. I desperately try to wipe my eyes and face clean, to try to slow things down, to find some calm. It's not at all effective. I take a couple of steps back to sit at the edge of my bed. I'm bent over, racked with sobs. Tears and snot and spit are falling from my face to the floor. I don't care.

I don't know how long this goes on. Long enough for my shoulders to start to ache and my stomach to feel as though I've done sit-ups for an hour. Everything still hurts. I can't breathe through my nose. I wipe my face clean with a corner of my blanket before I decide to crawl underneath it, working my way up into my bed. I lie down on my side. I've pulled my arms in tight to my chest, my knees tucked up as far as I can bring them.

"It's going to be okay," I whisper to myself, repeatedly, until my muscles finally begin to relax and the exhaustion of the day pulls me into a deep and restful and dreamless sleep.

✳ ✳ ✳

It's easier to push past your fears when you have somebody telling you what to do. No time to think, no time to react. Just do what they tell you to do. From Cindy helping me into the wheelchair that brought me to the operating room, to the new nurses here telling me where to go, that I should lie down here, my neurologists reminding me that there's nothing to worry about there, just rest and relax and take it easy — all I've needed to do is follow directions.

By now my part in all of this is dead simple. The hard work of this surgery falls squarely on the shoulders of the many other people in scrubs and face masks and thin plastic gloves milling about in this brightly lit room with me.

Now it's the anesthesiologist telling me to count down from one hundred. That's easy. That's an easy thing to do, just starting at ninety-nine, then ninety-eight and ninety-seven, before I start to get bored and think about what exactly it is that the neurologists will be doing. They'd explained it countless times, I know, using precision tools to cut a precise hole directly above one of the abscesses that had fortunately formed on the *surface* of my brain. The others were all over the place. Inside, behind my right eye, who knows where. This one, though, they've been able to map out with the MRIs and so they know exactly where to go. They're probably beaming a projection of my brain on my head. It's like a treasure map, with a big "X" marking the spot.

I think they have to use measuring tape to mark it with a Sharpie on my head. I'm already bald, so that part is a piece of cake. It might not be a tape measure, though? One of those soft ruler things, maybe, like when you're getting fitted for a suit? I forget what they call it. But, you know, it's probably that, because my head is round.

But they're not digging for treasure! They're not going to use shovels, of course. That's *ridiculous*. It's some kind of a drill. You know, like we used to have in wood shop in Mr. Eide's class in middle school, the old-fashioned kind where you've got one hand on top and another hand in the middle where there's this kind of crank, and that hand is cranking while the other hand is holding and then you're able to drill though anything! But it could be a power drill. I don't know. I'm not the doctor. They have all sorts of high-tech technology available to the doctors so I'm sure they'll use what they need.

And then, they'll take a cotton swab. Just like you use to clean out your ears. Same difference. It's just a thing you dab into the hole because the abscess is on top and you just want to dab it. To find out what it is. You've got, like, a petri dish next to you on the table. Not the operating table, because that's where I am. It's a different table that super sanitized. They power washed it, my neurologists, or wiped it down with Pledge. They cleaned, it okay, so the clean dish on the clean table is all ready for the sample that's on the cotton swab. The sample is the important part. It's the part where they'll know what kind of infection it is. That's the whole reason we're doing this right now.

Okay? Okay.

So I'm thinking there might be a problem.

I'm seeing that there's light around me again, and my eyes are still sensitive so it's tough to see, but I'm in this kind of a hallway with blankets and everything keeping me warm. I'm pretty sure that the brain surgeons were supposed to close up when they were done. Like put a cork or something into the hole in my head. No, not a cork. That's stupid. It would get wet and expand. A cork would never work. It's probably more like a cast I got when I'd broken my arm. They just put my head in that cast.

But here's the problem: if I'm in a hallway outside somewhere, then they're obviously done with my brain surgery. Except the top of my head feels ice cold. It feels like there's air on it. So I'm worried that they forgot to close my head when they got done. I'm afraid to touch up there. I don't want my brain to get any more infected than it already is.

Finally, a nurse comes through the hallway and I manage to make my mouth work to say words to her. "I think they forgot to close my brain," I tell her.

"I'm sorry. Your *what*?" she asks.

I start to yell at her. "My brain! My brains are still open!"

"No, no. You're okay," she says, contrary to all available evidence. It's *my* head. Does she think I don't know what it feels like to have my brain exposed to all these germs? If she's not going to listen, then I'm just going to take this pillow and cover up the hole in my head so my brains don't accidentally spill out.

What is this, fucking amateur hour? Do I have to do everything myself? It's impossible to stay awake so I fall asleep with my arms over the pillow over my head – the only one in this entire hospital who is responsible enough to keep my brains in place, apparently.

CHAPTER 35

I t works. Whatever they'd needed to find, they found. My stack of antibiotics is reduced to only two very specific, very targeted bags that appear to be doing a bang-up job. Penicillin is one of those. My counts have started to come back, too, which also helps. Fevers subside. My eye feels better. Not by much, mind you, but I'll take steps in a positive direction any day.

Shortly after surgery I end up arguing, unsuccessfully, with my neurologists.

Don't get me wrong. I'm super thankful, super grateful, can't express enough how happy I am for their brilliance and their deft touch. As near as any of us can tell, I'm still the same me. So that's fan-fucking-tastic. *However.*

My neurologist has prescribed something for me that I do not agree with. It's called Dilantin. An anti-seizure medication. It is absolutely standard, he explains, whenever a patient has had significant head trauma.

"But, that's not me," I say.

"You just had brain surgery," he answers.

"That's not *traumatic*, though."

"It is. It is literally how we define 'head trauma.'"

The problem with this isn't so much the definition but the prescription: he'd explained that Dilantin has several known side effects, one of which might make a patient's blood counts drop. That concerns me. Anything that might cause my blood counts to drop concerns me. I don't want to take the Dilantin. It is a losing argument.

Another losing argument in these dwindling summer days? I will not be going back to Carleton for fall term of my senior year. I've been thinking through how best to make it happen, trying to talk myself up that I'll be fine by then, no worries, but there are legitimate issues with logistics that can't be ignored. I've brought my wall calendar over to my bed multiple times, tapping my finger on the empty dates at the end of the month, and I can't figure out how to make it work. Dr. Collins has been cautiously optimistic about my departure date. Assuming my counts keep coming back the way they have been, and the abscesses continue to respond well to the fine-tuned antibiotics, then she expects I'll be good to go home sometime on or around August 20th. Labor Day is September third, meaning I'd want to fly to Minnesota on maybe the first or second of September? Dorms open on Sunday.

Best case, then, is I'd have only two weeks at home before returning to Carleton for a full load of classes. And I'm not nearly at full strength yet. Dr. Collins has told me that she wants me to come in once a week for blood draws after I leave. This is especially important with the Dilantin I've been taking. I wouldn't be surprised if she wants to schedule some additional CT scans or MRIs within the next month or so, too. All of that can be done at the Mayo Clinic in Rochester, of course, but it might be a bit aggressive for me to travel halfway across the country when we still need to keep such a close eye on my counts.

I'm also going to need to keep a steady supply of penicillin pumping into my body to make sure those abscesses never come back. There will be shipments coming to the house in Renton even before I leave. It'll be up to me to swap out my own bags. Not sure yet what I'm going to do without my little buddy around to hold everything, but I'll figure something out. Gravity works to control the flow of liquid down a tube that winds its way into my chest. Cindy had shown me an example of a small battery-powered pump that I can use for short periods of time if I want to get out of the house every now and then. Between what I'm hearing from her and confirming with Anne, the expectation is that I'll need to stay on that for at least six to eight weeks.

The operating phrase when treating these abscesses is "better safe than sorry." Any one of these obstacles are not insurmountable. Taken together, though, it's impossible to consider that I'll be able to start my senior year in September. Better safe than sorry, right?

This is so incredibly disappointing. Getting back to school has been my primary goal for so much of my hospitalization. It's difficult to let go of that dream, so close to the finish. It sucks, is what it does. *Stupid fucking leukemia. When are you going to stop screwing up everything?*

I talk with Mom about it first, then Dad and Jane, trying to be all rational and precise with my explanations. I realize — twice — that my family has been so supportive of me wanting to return to Northfield for my senior year because they knew how important it was for me, not because they actually wanted it to happen. They'd been worried about logistics, too, but were prepared to support whatever decision I'd made. There is palpable relief on everybody's faces when I tell them that I think it's best if I stay at home this fall. This final round of chemo was much tougher than any of us expected. There's no sense in making this next period of recovery that much more difficult by pushing too fast for a goal that was probably out of reach before I'd even started my first round of chemo back in March.

It's settled, then: Carleton will have to wait until winter term. But at least I'll be home soon. *For good!* That's the best possible news, overshadowing, by far, the disappointment I've been feeling.

* * *

I don't have much fight in me when I get home this time. I'm so tired. I know that I'm done with the University of Washington Medical Center, so I don't feel the need to get out for runs, to drop to the floor when I'm watching Regis and Kathie Lee in the morning, banging out ten or twenty push-ups during the commercial breaks.

I miss Cindy, of course. I miss Anne. I miss our routine. The last day or two before I'd gotten the okay to go home was this confusing mix of happiness and sadness. I didn't know it was possible to feel two polar opposites at the same time. I am so happy to be out of that fucking place. And yet, I am so grateful, so thankful that I was able to get through everything, something I know wouldn't have been possible without the steady hands of Cindy and Anne, and a part of me wishes I could stay.

I don't think about this. As soon as I do, the tears start up again. No time for that. So let's just not think about it, okay? I'm happy to be home and I miss the company of my two nurses and that's all. I'd hugged them both before I'd left. I'd thanked them, then. That's enough, isn't it?

My new routine is quiet. I'm not mad at cancer. I'm not angry at the world. Scott and Blake keep wanting to take me out clubbing, or bar hopping in Pioneer Square. I tell them I'm not interested. It has nothing to do with the scar on my head. I'm tired. I hope they understand.

Blake and I haven't spoken about what I'd said to him before my brain surgery. I tried, one night when he'd stopped by the house to see if I wanted to grab a bite to eat. He shook his head when I started to apologize, cutting me off with a wave of his hand.

"It's okay," he'd said. "I know. We're good."

I roll out of bed each morning, still wearing the pajamas that Gail had bought for me back in the beginning. The hardwood floors at home are cold on my feet. I'll pour a bowl of cereal, a glass of OJ, and bring both to the living room. Paul had screwed a hook into the ceiling before I came home. Something you might use to hang a potted fern or something. I reach into the cardboard box that's on the floor, up against the couch, and take out a new bag of penicillin. It goes above me. The dial on my tube is blue. I don't really need to adjust it anymore, but I do anyway. The drops of penicillin shouldn't come down too fast. I'm able to eyeball it by now.

Kathie Lee is talking about Coda. He's such a cute baby! I'll eat my cereal and drink my juice and then my legs come up onto the couch, resting my head on a cushion while I watch the TV sideways. I'm still so tired. It's okay, though. Tired at home is better than tired anywhere else.

✳ ✳ ✳

Near the end of the month, Blake drives me up to the hospital to get my counts checked. They are well below normal. Dr. Collins doesn't want me to leave the hospital, so I get my fourth room at the UWMC. Still on the opposite side, no view of the Cascades, just the gloom of early October.

Dilantin is the likely culprit. Of course that's what it has to be. Chekov's fucking gun, right? Dr. Collins cuts it from my regular course of meds. Now I'm only getting penicillin, still, hopefully for not much longer. She wants to keep me here under observation to confirm her theory.

Cindy wakes me harshly the next morning. She's angry with me. "What are you doing here?" She tries to pull me out of the bed, joking, I think, but maybe not, trying to kick me out of the room. "You weren't supposed to come back!" she yells.

As expected, my counts recover by the end of the week. Cindy and Anne and I have a lot of time to talk. No fevers. No headaches. No unexpected bleeding. I'm hungry all the time. I'm an infinitely easier patient, now, than I've ever been.

We say our goodbyes, again, one last time.

CHAPTER 36

The rest of the year passes by quickly. Weekly visits to the UWMC result in nothing but nothing. Blood counts continue to look as steady as if I'd never had leukemia or chemo or anything. MRI's are pristine. Dr. Collins finally tells me I can stop the penicillin, which frees me to go out at night without needing to carry my small fanny-pack pump. The penicillin was also the only reason I've needed to keep my Hickman catheter, so she removes that, too. Everything is easier now. Simple.

I settle into a similar routine as what I'd had during the summer: eat as much as I can, sleep as much as I can, work out, run, yell at leukemia when my weakened legs struggle up a hill, spend nearly every weekend with Scott and Blake and Jeff. My hair has grown back, just barely. It's short enough to look like an intentional decision to go with a buzz cut, like I'd done for most of my senior year in high school. Still long enough, though, to cover the small horseshoe-shaped scar on top of my head. My fingers run lazily along the edges of the scar, tracing it back and forth during my many quiet moments. My vision returns to normal.

There's time to reflect, now. To think. But I don't want to. My friends and I will go out on weekends, still, to the same familiar places. It's nice to be back to normal. It's great to get out and not worry about anything. There's nothing to see here: I'm just an average, every-day, normal twenty-one-year-old college kid out with his best friends for an evening of fun and entertainment.

The days continue to get colder and darker and wetter through November and December. I'm excited for what the new year will bring. I can't wait to put 1990 behind me.

A letter arrives from Lancaster: it's from Colin Lyas, addressed to both Mom and me. I quickly tear it open. Colin wishes me well. He knows it's been a little while since he's written, which he apologizes for, and says he's glad to hear — via the Off-Campus Studies office at Carleton — that I'll be returning there to finish my studies. He's happy to know that things have progressed well since I'd left Lancaster.

He apologizes again for not having written sooner, but it had all happened so fast. Rosemary's lung cancer diagnosis had surprised both of them, and he'd found himself returning to the same hallways at the Royal Lancaster Infirmary he'd visited when they'd said their goodbyes to me in late February. And the cancer took her from him too soon, he writes. She was only fifty-one, full of vigor, and the unequivocal love of his life. He wasn't sure what he would be doing next, if he'd stay in Lancaster or not. He wanted Mom to know that he valued the short time that they'd spent together, all of them, drinking wine, smoking cigarettes, eating paella that Rosemary had prepared on a cold winter night at their home in Lancaster.

The letter closes with Colin once more wishing me well, for my return to Carleton and all the happy, healthy years to follow.

EPILOGUE

This is where the "happily ever after" is supposed to come, the boundless epiphanies about the importance of embracing life, where with a bolt of lightning your narrator is forever changed and it's all rainbows and unicorns and seizing the day. Only that's not how it happened. I could write an entire book to talk about how much that didn't happen for me.

I learned how to survive. I would put one foot in front of the other, no matter how bad things got, pushing ahead to get to tomorrow. I learned that if you can make it through any day then you can make it through every day. That attitude enabled me to almost immediately pretend that nothing bad had really happened. Hair grows back and weight returns and pretty soon there's no discernible difference between who I was before leukemia and who I'd become after. So where's the harm in desperately searching for as much normalcy as I could possibly find?

There's nothing wrong with me. I had leukemia, okay? Past tense. Now back off. Leave me the fuck alone so I can get on with living my perfectly normal perfectly pristine perfectly mundane life.

It took me a very, very long time to begin to appreciate how lucky I'd been. That low, steady hum of leukemia – those palpable memories that were so painfully fresh the first few years after I left the hospital for the final time – slowly transformed into quiet background noise. The early anger subsided. It settled down. I was able to reflect on the spring and summer and fall of 1990 and appreciate how fortunate I'd been to make it through without any lasting complications or long-term consequences. As much as I wanted leukemia to be nothing more than a brutal speed bump on the way to the rest of my life, I began to understand that while I didn't have to let the experience define me, it would always be an important part of me.

But perhaps I'm getting ahead of myself. Those are some painful lessons learned after any number of bumps and bruises along the way. It's almost easy, I suppose, to focus on the finish line when you're dealing with leukemia. The numbers don't lie. You either have cancer or you don't, and as long as you still do you're going to have to do your best with what your doctors tell you, trusting the process, dealing with side effects, not letting your mind wander too much when you're beginning to lose hope.

I got through. I was somehow able to weather any number of storms to survive a form of leukemia that most people do not. There is no magic formula, no secret to my success. Any of the things that made a difference for me – being surrounded by loving friends and family, a positive attitude, unbelievably skilled and compassionate nurses, determination, perseverance, dumb luck – don't guarantee anything for anybody.

I had leukemia, okay? I had it and now I don't and I'm glad that's not the end of my story. I am grateful, every day, for the extra chances I've been given to remain alive on this planet, grateful for two beautiful, brilliant, talented daughters – now around the same age as I was when my doctors couldn't say for sure if I'd ever be able to have children after the potent mix of toxic chemicals they'd be using to save my life.

I am grateful that I was finally able to figure out that life is meant to be enjoyed, not endured, a lesson I'm still learning every day.

ABOUT THE AUTHOR

I was born and raised in Renton, Washington – a suburb just south of Seattle – before heading off to Carleton College in Minnesota. All things considered, I've been exceptionally lucky in the years since leukemia turned everything upside-down during my junior year in Lancaster, England.

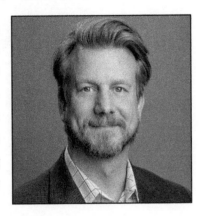

There have been remarkable amounts of normalcy punctuated by some highlights: the only times I've spent the night in a hospital since 1990 was when my daughters, Esmé and Jasmine, were born. They're both currently pursuing their dreams on opposite coasts. It's impossible to describe how fortunate I am to be their father.

It took me a *long* time to understand how to express my gratitude, mostly in a variety of ways that push me well outside my comfort zone: a handful of marathons with Team in Training, and any number of other regular fundraising efforts for *The Leukemia and Lymphoma Society*. For good or bad, directly or indirectly, cancer changes the lives of everyone it touches. It's what we choose to do with that change that makes all the difference.

CPSIA information can be obtained
at www.ICGtesting.com
Printed in the USA
LVHW032228180220
647337LV00005B/688

9 781733 159005